TOO FLEXIBLE TO FEEL GOOD

A PRACTICAL ROADMAP TO MANAGING HYPERMOBILITY

Celest PEREIRA & **Adell BRIDGES**

VICTORY BELT PUBLISHING
Las Vegas

First published in 2021 by Victory Belt Publishing, Inc.

Copyright © 2021 Celest Pereira and Adell Bridges

ISBN-13: 978-1-628604-17-7

The information included in this book is for educational purposes only. It is not intended or implied to be a substitute for professional medical advice. The reader should always consult their healthcare provider to determine the appropriateness of the information for their own situation or if they have questions regarding a medical condition or treatment plan. The statements in this book have not been evaluated by the Food and Drug Administration, nor are they intended to diagnose, treat, cure, or prevent any disease. The authors and publisher expressly disclaim responsibility for any adverse effects that may result from the use or application of the information contained in this book.

Cover and interior design and illustrations by Yordan Terziev and Boryana Yordanova

Printed in Canada
TC 0222

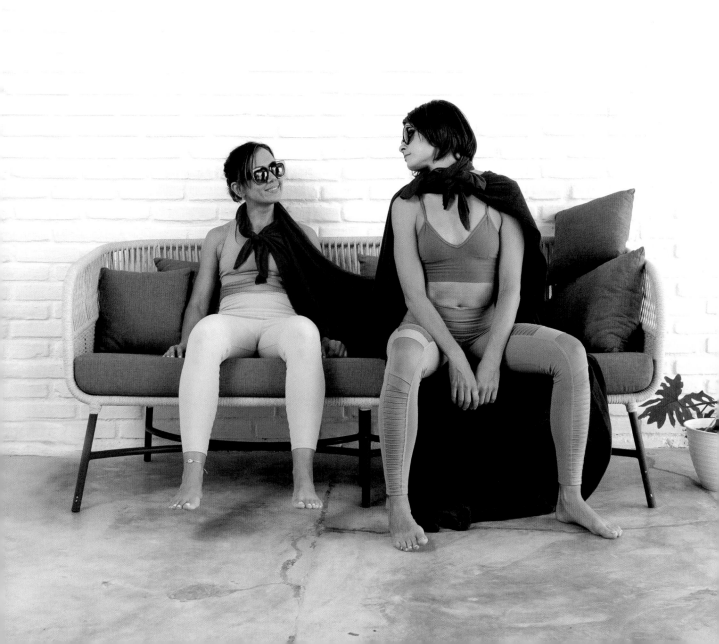

TABLE OF CONTENTS

FOREWORD

My name is Dr. Eric Cobb, and I am the founder of Z-Health Performance—an education company that specializes in what we call brain-based or neurocentric training. Put simply, our company has spent two decades trying to bring the brain into the world of health, fitness, pain relief, and rehabilitation. Our primary job is helping professionals make the shift from a biomechanical approach to viewing the body and movement through a neurobiomechanical lens.

During this time, I've met and worked with thousands of amazing individuals—doctors, therapists, researchers, coaches, athletes, and more from all over the world. While I've learned so much from so many of them, it has been rare to meet professionals who have such a vision for helping their clients that they are willing to learn, grow, and change a model that has already been successful. This is one of the reasons it gives me such tremendous pleasure to be asked to write this foreword for Celest and Adell.

Just over a year ago, I was introduced to these two wonderful people via the wonders of Instagram. While I am a bit of a Luddite when it comes to social media because of the tremendous amount of misinformation sent out to the world on an hourly basis, it can still be a powerful force for good.

My first introduction to their work occurred via their Hypermobile Yogis account. I was immediately drawn to some of the photos and content because they were directly echoing so much of what we know about hypermobility. Their side-by-side photographs demonstrating "decreased" flexibility coupled with their focus on these changes as a better result of training sparked the desire to learn more about their approach. This led to a yearlong whirlwind exchange of ideas regarding bringing neurology more deeply into their already fantastic work.

Here's why this matters.

As a neurology guy, I have an intense interest in noticeable differences in brain function and structure in different populations. Having a background of working with professional dancers and world-class gymnasts, I had already invested quite a lot of time digging into the existing research around hypermobility and the brain.

As it turns out, we already know a lot, and it's incredibly fascinating. The simple takeaway is that the hypermobile brain is different, and the differences matter not just in terms of movement, but also in fatigue, pain, anxiety, and a host of other issues. The question has been, like so much research, how can we take this information and make it practical?

In this book, you are going to find some critical answers to that question. While some of the material may seem a bit strange at first, rest assured that it is based both on credible research and real-world application.

The hypermobile population has long been underserved or ignored in traditional training approaches. This is incredibly unfortunate because, as I mentioned, research is clearly demonstrating that hypermobile brains are different. This means that a specific, targeted training program is essential for making these bendy bodies as pain-free and functional as possible.

Celest and Adell have done a remarkable job over the last year of studying brain-based training concepts and integrating them into their own personal training and coaching with tremendous results. I am so pleased to see them incorporating these concepts into this book and so excited to hear about the life-changing results you will experience as you apply them in your own training.

Keep Moving,

Dr. Eric Cobb
Founder, Z-Health Performance

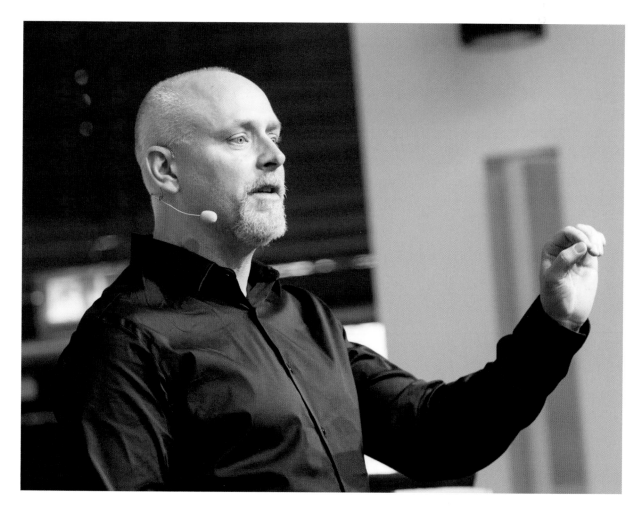

INTRODUCTION

There are superhumans among us, and you may be one of them. On the surface, these people seem to be less-than-ordinary living wrecks. They are marooned with fatigue while others around them are power-boating with seemingly never-ending energy. They have ongoing gut issues even after years of obsessive attention to healthy eating, more than any of their "I-give-birth-once-a-day-to-a-perfectly-formed-poop" friends. They are secret heroes who somehow cope with stomach-churning anxiety even though they have a brimming personal arsenal of meditation and breathing techniques to help spawn some semblance of calm and inner peace.

Often, they are made to feel, by their doctors, their peers, and the rest of society, like hypochondriacs or freaks, when in truth they are unknowingly walking around with untapped superhuman abilities.

We're talking about people with joint hypermobility spectrum disorder (JHSD or hypermobility for short), and the reasons they (and perhaps you too) are superhuman will become clear as you work your way through this book. For now, know that if you picked up this book because you thought, *"Too Flexible to Feel Good?* That sounds like me!" you are not imagining your symptoms. You're not a freak, you're not a hypochondriac, and you are definitely not alone.

WHAT IS HYPERMOBILITY?

Hypermobility is a spectrum disorder that affects around 15 to 20 percent of the population, meaning it's more common than being left-handed, standing over six feet tall, or having a third nipple.[1] (It's difficult to know precisely how many people are affected since hypermobility so often goes undiagnosed and indeed unnoticed.) Therefore, it may seem baffling that you can bring it up at any dinner party, maybe even a dinner party full of doctors, and hear most of them say, "Wow, I've never heard of it!" (The sheer lack of awareness of this disorder sends shivers down our spines.)

One reason for this is that the spectrum nature of the disorder makes it challenging to spot. It's not exactly a third nipple, right there for you to see in all its glory every time you look in the mirror. Also, a spectrum disorder has minimal effects on some people, allowing them to lead normal healthy lives, whereas others can be ticking time bombs of chronic illness, struggling with eclectic arrays of symptoms that, frankly, suck ass.

A MOMENT TO GROVEL TO THE EDS SUPERHEROES

These incredible superhumans who find themselves on the far end of the spectrum, where the condition can be debilitating, have what is known as Ehlers-Danlos Syndrome (EDS). EDS is a very complex condition, and going into the details of it is beyond the scope of this book. However, we would like to take this opportunity to acknowledge all our friends with EDS for being incredibly brave, as they face immense challenges in daily life.

EDS is a genetic mutation that takes stretchy issues to epic new proportions. These heroes face frequent joint dislocations and fractures, frequent bruising, problems with their organs and blood vessels, fragile eyes, and breathing problems, to name but a few of the issues EDS can cause.[2] Before we move on, we'd like to say to all our readers with EDS that we apologize for not giving EDS the attention it deserves. Perhaps, if this book is well received, we will get funding to write a book just for this neglected community.

After much digging, most people with JHSD unearth the fact that they exist somewhere along the spectrum. Some are a little confused by their unusual symptoms, while others are downright tearing their hair out from sheer frustration at the mountain of medical bills.

So what do these people on the sliding scale of hypermobility look like? Are you one of them? How do you know? How do you spot one if you're a yoga teacher, dance instructor, or sports coach and want to keep your clients safe from injury?

Well, first off, we think *hypermobility* is a misnomer. We personally believe this condition should be known as joint hyper*flexibility* spectrum disorder. The most obvious trait that our flexible family present with is—you guessed it—*super flexibility*.[3] Often (but not always), their knees and elbows hyperextend (go beyond 180 degrees). They may be able to dislocate their shoulders as a party trick. They can fold themselves like origami while sitting on the floor playing a board game. During yoga, they can put their heads in places heads should never go. Fingers can bend backward when innocently picking a nose.

We will cover the range of other symptoms that come along with all the seemingly impressive bending later. For now, one thing is a fact: our Bendy Family are either progressively drifting further toward the worsening edge of the scale, *or* they are taking the steps needed to see massive improvements in their bodies. There is no standing still on the scale; you're either improving or deconditioning.

We created this book for hypermobile people who want to harness their stretchy powers and go beyond just managing their symptoms. We have dubbed those with JHSD "Bendy People" or our "Bendy Family," and they are the protagonists and heroes of this story. For they are *[cue cinematic music]* **superhumans** (in training).

MEET ADELL AND CELEST

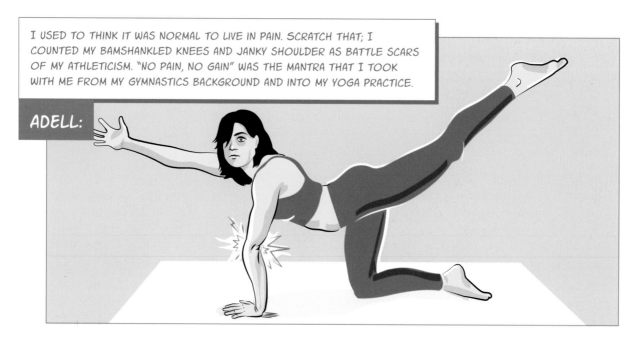

I USED TO THINK IT WAS NORMAL TO LIVE IN PAIN. SCRATCH THAT; I COUNTED MY BAMSHANKLED KNEES AND JANKY SHOULDER AS BATTLE SCARS OF MY ATHLETICISM. "NO PAIN, NO GAIN" WAS THE MANTRA THAT I TOOK WITH ME FROM MY GYMNASTICS BACKGROUND AND INTO MY YOGA PRACTICE.

ADELL:

YOGA BECAME BOTH A COMPETITION ARENA FOR HOW DEEP I COULD PRETZEL MYSELF AND THE PLACE WHERE I LEARNED TO EXPERIENCE MY BODY IN A NEW WAY; I LEARNED TO LISTEN. GRANTED, I IGNORED WHAT I HEARD FROM MY BODY (WHIMPERING WITH PAIN AND BEGGING ME TO HOLD BACK).

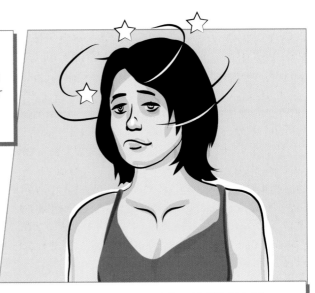

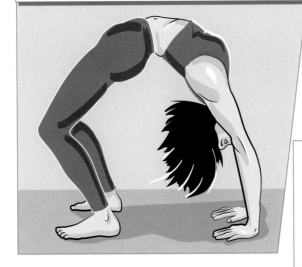

INSTEAD, I KEPT STRIVING TO KEEP THE "YOU'RE SO GOOD AT YOGA" PRAISE ROLLING IN WHILE IGNORING THE GROWING LIST OF ANNOYING BUT NOT LIFE-THREATENING ISSUES CREEPING INTO MY DAILY LIFE, FROM UNEXPLAINED BOUTS OF CRIPPLING FATIGUE TO WEIRD DIGESTIVE PROBLEMS THAT MY FRIENDS DIDN'T SEEM TO HAVE TO DEAL WITH, AND THAT MY DOCTORS DISMISSED.

AT MY YOGA TEACHER TRAINING, I WAS LUCKILY INFECTED WITH ANATOMY GEEKITIS AND BECAME THE WORLD'S TOP GOOGLER FOR EVERY TYPE OF MOVEMENT IMAGINABLE. ONE DAY, A GOOGLE SEARCH FOR SOMETHING I CAN'T REMEMBER NOW--PROBABLY "HOW TO GET AN OVERSPLIT" OR "STRETCHES FOR DEEPER BACKBENDS"--LED ME DOWN THE RABBIT HOLE OF JOINT HYPERMOBILITY. AS I READ THROUGH THE SYMPTOMS, I FELT LIKE I WAS GOING THROUGH A CHECKLIST OF ISSUES THAT I THOUGHT WERE JUST NORMAL LIFE.

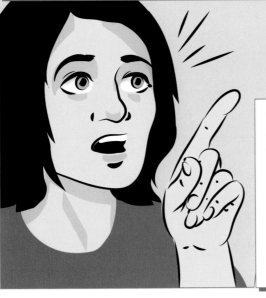

I WISH I COULD SAY THAT I UNDERSTOOD STRAIGHTAWAY EVERYTHING I NEEDED TO DO DIFFERENTLY IN MY LIFE AND IN MY YOGA PRACTICE TO ALLEVIATE ALL MY SYMPTOMS, BUT A MIXTURE OF IGNORANCE OF BIOMECHANICS AND AN ATTACHMENT TO THE WAY I WAS DOING THINGS MEANT THAT I STILL HAD A LONG JOURNEY AHEAD OF ME. SUFFICE IT TO SAY THAT I'M STILL ON THAT JOURNEY. OVER TIME, THOUGH, RELUCTANCE TO ALTER MY YOGA PRACTICE TURNED TO ENTHUSIASM AS I EXPERIENCED HOW SUPERHUMAN IT FELT TO COMBINE MY HYPERFLEXIBILITY AND HYPERSENSITIVITY WITH STRENGTH AND STABILITY.

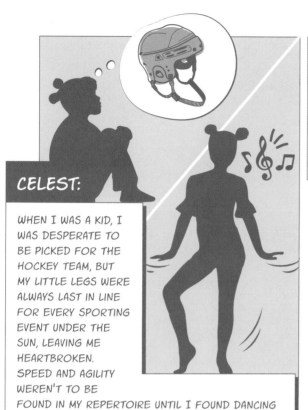

CELEST:

WHEN I WAS A KID, I WAS DESPERATE TO BE PICKED FOR THE HOCKEY TEAM, BUT MY LITTLE LEGS WERE ALWAYS LAST IN LINE FOR EVERY SPORTING EVENT UNDER THE SUN, LEAVING ME HEARTBROKEN. SPEED AND AGILITY WEREN'T TO BE FOUND IN MY REPERTOIRE UNTIL I FOUND DANCING AS A HOBBY. FINALLY I HAD A MOVEMENT OUTLET THAT DIDN'T CARE HOW TALL I WAS AND LOVED THE FACT THAT I WAS BENDY AF.

HOWEVER, AS A CHILD AND YOUNG ADULT, I STRUGGLED WITH A CONSTANT BARRAGE OF PAIN, FROM THE OBVIOUS INJURIES TO RANDOM UNEXPLAINED ACHES. MY GUT ISSUES WERE SEVERE, OFTEN LEAVING ME SHOOTING TO THE LOO IN THE MIDDLE OF GROCERY SHOPPING. AND OFTEN I HAD TO COPE WITH MY HEART RACING FROM ANXIETY AS A RESPONSE TO STRESSES BIG AND SMALL.

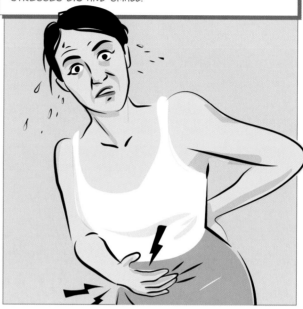

WHILE STUDYING FOR MY PHYSIOTHERAPY DEGREE, I LEARNED ABOUT HYPERMOBILITY, BUT I STILL DIDN'T MAKE THE CONNECTION IN MY OWN BODY. IT WASN'T UNTIL YOGA USHERED ME OFF TO THE PHYSIOTHERAPIST CLINIC WITH DEBILITATING INJURIES. EVEN THOUGH MY BODY WAS CRYING OUT FOR CHANGE, MY EGO WOULD ALWAYS OVERRULE IN THE HOPE THAT I COULD GET INSTAGRAM LIKES FOR BEING "AMAZING." AFTER NUMEROUS VISITS TO THE PHYSIOTHERAPIST, I WAS AT LAST DIAGNOSED WITH HYPERMOBILITY, AND IT WAS THIS DIAGNOSIS THAT HELPED ME SEEK OUT SAFE ADAPTATIONS TO MY YOGA PRACTICE.

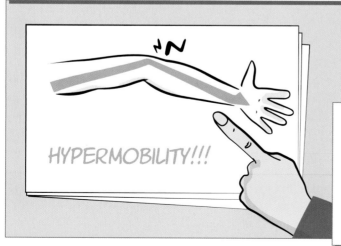

HYPERMOBILITY!!!

AFTER MAKING DRASTIC CHANGES IN MY PRACTICE AND FEELING THE POSITIVE EFFECTS IN MY BODY, I WAS HEARTBROKEN TO SEE MY YOGA PEERS PUSHING THROUGH PAIN TO ACHIEVE DEEPER POSES.

SOME USEFUL WORDS TO KNOW

ROM: Our term of endearment for range of motion. (Or maybe it's just the initials.) Range of motion refers to how far a joint can move in any given direction. We'll discuss it in more depth in Chapter 1 on the nervous system as well as in Chapter 10, the Bendy Person's Yoga Survival Kit.

Mobility: Range of motion, specifically the useful type. As in, the ability to move a body part with control.

One way to think about mobility is as a combination of flexibility and strength. Bendy People often have little strength, and their ability to move into impressive pretzel poses or postures is reliant on an outside force such as gravity or an assisting hand or prop to grab and pull.[4] Think of someone with both feet up on chairs and their hips resting on the floor in an oversplit, thanks only to gravity and no strength in their leg muscles. If the chairs were removed, this person's legs would fall without control to the earth.

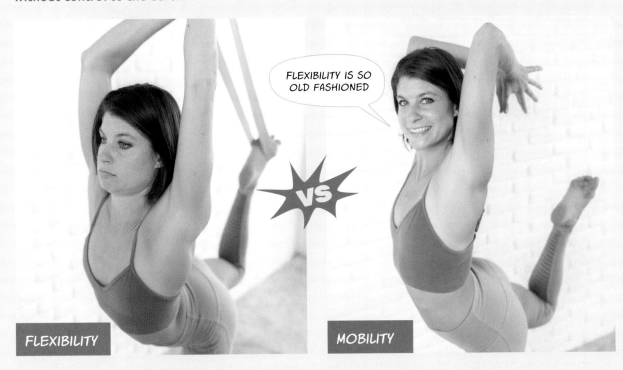

FLEXIBILITY IS SO OLD FASHIONED

VS

FLEXIBILITY

MOBILITY

Collagen: The most abundant protein in the body and the main structure of the fascia and soft tissues such as muscles, tendons, and ligaments, as well as the gut lining, the walls of the arteries, and the skin.[5] Most relevant for this book, a disruption of collagen is the cause of JHSD. It is because the structure of the collagen is, basically, extra stretchy that Bendy People are so flexible.[3]

Tension: In the context of this book, tension is the ability of a bodily structure to hold its shape. The greater the tension, the greater the potential energy that can be stored within it.[6] Think of a rubber band versus a bungee cord. You could easily hold a rubber band on either end and pull it apart because it holds almost no tension. A bungee cord would be much harder to stretch out using just your arms. But hang a heavy object (maybe you, you daredevil) from one end of a rubber band, and it will snap, whereas the bungee cord will allow the daring bungee-er to bounce back up safely. Boing! We need this kind of tension in our bodies to hold our bodily structures together.

WHY PEOPLE ARE HYPERMOBILE

You may have noticed in the sidebar on the previous page that collagen is an ingredient in more than just the body parts that affect range of motion. Yes, Bendy People also often have hyperflexible blood vessels, extra-stretchy skin, and a digestive tract that may lack the tension it needs to do its job properly.

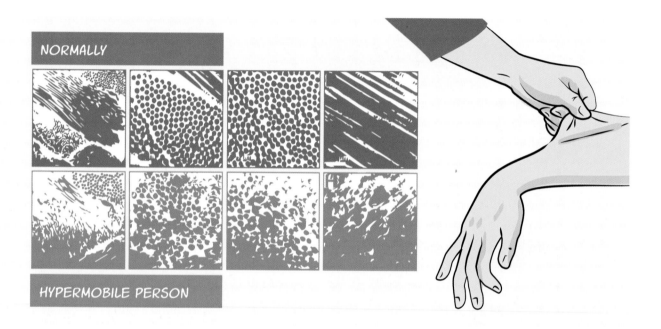

NORMALLY

HYPERMOBILE PERSON

The reason is a disruption of how the collagen is organized, which can affect some or all areas of the body, depending on the severity of the diagnosis. Sadly, that doesn't mean just the muscles and connective tissues of the body (aka the myofascial system). Nope; hypermobility often (but not always) comes with a higher rate of gut and digestive issues such as irritable bowel syndrome (IBS), acid reflux, and constipation. Bendy People suffer from a higher rate of anxiety than the average population.[7] Fatigue is another common symptom. Asthma, migraines, fibromyalgia, postural orthostatic tachycardia syndrome (POTS), hypotension, insomnia, prolapse, cystitis, hemorrhoids, varicose veins, and more irritating issues are seen in higher proportions among our Bendy Family.[8]

On the plus side, we also suffer from less atherosclerosis, and giving birth is generally a bit easier...a bit. It's still childbirth, after all, but it is theorized that having stretchy tissues can alleviate the discomfort of passing a human baby through your fanny.[9]

Don't fall into the trap of thinking that you or someone you know is hypermobile just because you have a couple of these conditions. They simply occur *at higher rates* among the Bendy population.

Enter the terribly-flawed-and-inconclusive-yet-still-the-best-thing-we've-got Beighton scale.

A spectrum disorder, which comes with symptoms that also affect members of the population who don't have the disorder, is a tricky thing. And so the Beighton scale is still in use today despite being far from scientific in its conclusiveness.[10]

Here's the test. You get one point for each thing you can do:

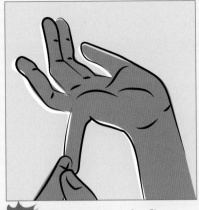

1 Your right pinky finger bends backward past 90 degrees.

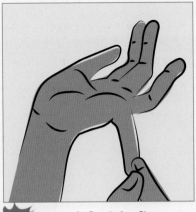

2 Your left pinky finger bends backward past 90 degrees.

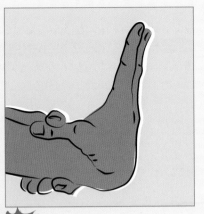

3 Your right wrist can be bent into flexion, allowing your thumb to touch your forearm.

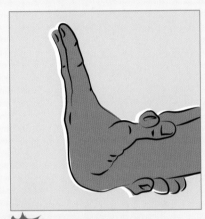

4 Your left wrist can be bent into flexion, allowing your thumb to touch your forearm.

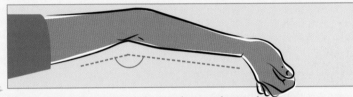

5 Your right elbow straightens beyond 180 degrees.

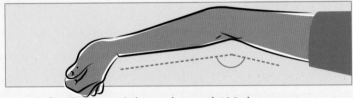

6 Your left elbow straightens beyond 180 degrees.

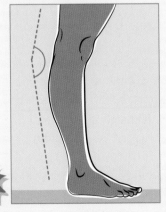

7 Your right knee straightens beyond 180 degrees.

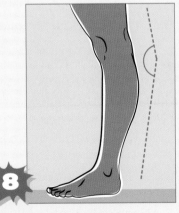

8 Your left knee straightens beyond 180 degrees.

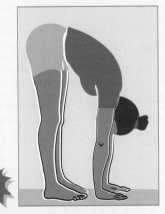

9 You can place your hands flat on the floor while standing with your knees straight.

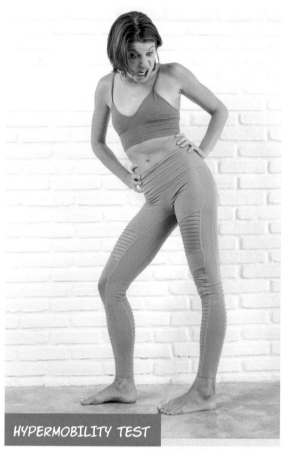

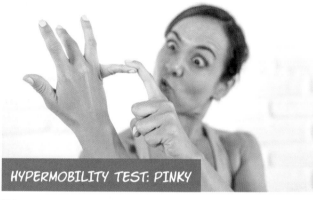

HYPERMOBILITY TEST: PINKY

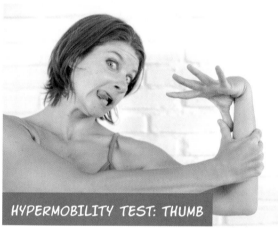

HYPERMOBILITY TEST: THUMB

HYPERMOBILITY TEST

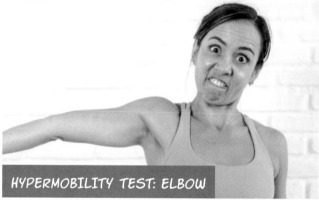

HYPERMOBILITY TEST: ELBOW

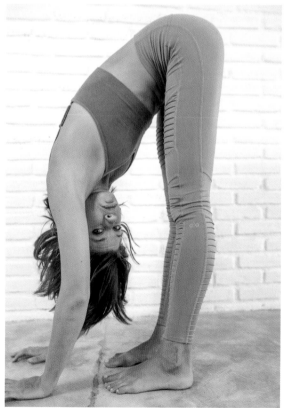

Some sources say you need to score only two points to be considered hypermobile. Others say you need four or five. So, who knows? Given that it's a spectrum disorder, perhaps even one point means you could be on the spectrum. The important thing is whether or not your abilities indicate that you have a condition that is causing you pain or putting you at risk of developing pain later in life.

That is exactly what this book is going to address. But first, let's talk about what hypermobility is *not*.

WHAT HYPERMOBILITY IS NOT

It's tempting to use a this-or-that mentality toward complex issues such as joint hypermobility. For sure, when we learn about a condition that affects us from head to toe and in all aspects of life, it's easy to want to blame everything on hypermobility at first. It's like discovering you have an intolerance to gluten and cutting gluten out of your diet. Your skin begins to glow, your energy levels improve, and you're not farting all the time. However, you wouldn't expect all the traffic lights to turn green for you or to get that promotion just because you stopped eating gluten. You know the difference between gut issues and life issues, and you know that they are often unrelated.

With hypermobility, it's even more complicated, because JHSD can affect the walls of your digestive organs, your blood vessels, your proprioception, your skin, *and* your ligaments, tendons, and muscles, and that leads to a very long list of things that have a positive correlation to JHSD— meaning there are more people with JHSD who have these conditions than people who aren't hypermobile.

But that doesn't mean gut issues make you hypermobile. It doesn't mean if you have anxiety, you're on the spectrum for joint hypermobility. It doesn't even mean that you're hypermobile if you're really flexible! Similarly, if you do have JHSD, it doesn't necessarily mean that your gut issues are related to the collagen disruption that causes your loosey-goosey joints. Maybe they are simply related to your diet or a strong round of antibiotics you took when you were a teenager.

Basically, you need to watch out for that little voice that wants to oversimplify a complex issue. Beware of any temptation to self-diagnose just because something sounds familiar.

To satisfy your craving for cold, hard facts, here are a few things that hypermobility is definitely, certainly, matter-of-factly *not:*

- A condition that means you're flexible *everywhere.* You might be, but chances are you have some "tight" areas of your body that are trying to offer protection.[11] (More on that in Chapter 2 on biomechanics.)

- A condition that affects only children and women. Yes, it's more common among children and women, but anybody, at any age, of any sex, can be hypermobile.[1]

- A condition that affects only the joints. As we'll discuss in later chapters, there are other things to deal with besides flexy knees and elbows.[2]

- Something that means you'll forever live in pain and that you can deal with only by taking painkillers. *T*he ignorance that has led to this belief gives us nightmares! *The horror! The horror!!*

- A condition that affects you alone, and nobody understands you or what you have to live with.

- A totally crappy condition with no benefits or positives. (Just a reminder: you're actually superhuman.)

- An explanation for being a total weirdo. Your weirdness is, rather, your beautiful ability to be uniquely yourself and not try to fit into any boxes or norms. Embrace it!

- An excuse to show people how easily you can dislocate your shoulder or put your leg over your head. Just because you *can* do it doesn't mean you *should.*

CHAPTER 1:

A TEENSY WEENSY LITTLE INTRODUCTION OF THE NERVOUS SYSTEM

To get the most out of this book, it's important to understand how the nervous system works and just how intimately linked it is with every single experience of your life.

Consider this: You don't see with your eyes; you see with your *brain.* Your eyes are just the equipment that gives your brain information from the outside world that your brain then interprets, leading you to have a greater awareness of what's in front of your face.[12]

You don't hear with your ears; they are just equipment. You hear with your *brain.*[13] You don't feel pain from a cut on your leg with the skin in that area; you feel the pain with your *brain.*[14]

Ever been dumped and left sobbing for days as you eat tubs of ice cream? You don't feel heartbreak in your heart; you feel it in your *brain.*[15]

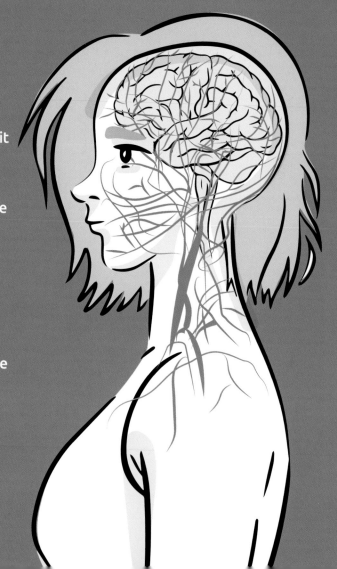

Finish these sentences:

I don't move with my muscles. I move with my _____.

I don't feel pain in my joints. I feel pain with my _____.

I don't taste that post-heartbreak-wallowing ice cream with my tongue. I taste it with my _____.

The brain is part of the central nervous system, and it communicates to the rest of the body through the peripheral nervous system. Think of the brain as a central hub with millions and millions of channels (nerves) running from it to send and receive signals to and from the rest of the body.[16]

Nothing happens without communication between the brain and the nervous system. Sometimes this communication is flawed. Sometimes it's murky and muddled. Sometimes it doesn't work altogether. Usually it works just fine, though, and that's something to be in awe of!

Before we go any further, we'd like to introduce you to Elastidog.

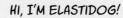

HI, I'M ELASTIDOG!

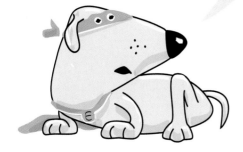

This is Elastidog, who is here to help us understand the nervous system, or at least the ways in which it applies to us Bendy Peeps and how we experience the world. No, the human nervous system is not a furry quadrupedal mammal, but it does share some similarities with Elastidog.

UNDERSTANDING NEURAL PATHWAYS

One very, very, very important trait to remember about the nervous system is that it is *adaptable*. It constantly uses what we call *neural pathways* to make our lives easier, and those neural pathways are constantly adapting.[17]

LAST NIGHT, ELASTIDOG'S HUMANS, MOLLY AND TOM, HAD A RACK OF RIBS FOR DINNER. MOLLY HAS TAUGHT ELASTIDOG THAT IF HE SITS NEXT TO HER AND WAITS FOR HER TO SAY,

TWIRL, ELASTIDOG! TWIRL!

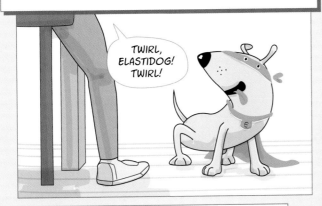

...THEN HE JUST HAS TO SPIN AROUND IN A CIRCLE AND MOLLY WILL GIVE HIM A BONE.

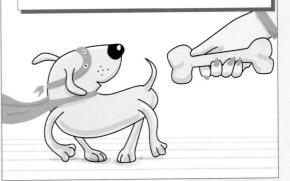

MOLLY WAS FEELING GENEROUS AND GAVE HIM TWO BONES, SO HE HID ONE AWAY FOR LATER, ALTHOUGH NOW HE CAN'T REMEMBER WHERE.

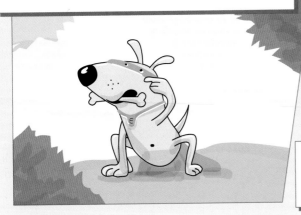

WHAT ELASTIDOG DOESN'T KNOW IS THAT A COUPLE OF MICE FOUND THE BONE AND CARRIED IT TO THEIR FAVORITE SNACKING SPOT UNDER THE OLD OAK TREE,

AND FROM THERE A FOX TOOK IT TO HAVE A NIBBLE WITH HER CUBS WHO WERE PLAYING IN THE MUD BY THE STREAM.

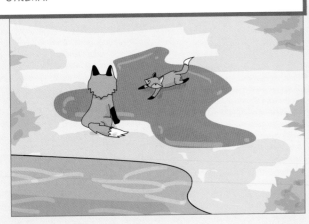

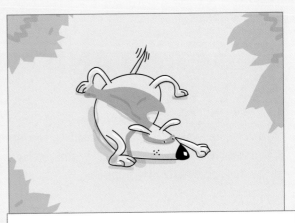

SO, AS ELASTIDOG SET OFF TO FIND HIS BONE, NOSE TO THE FLOOR, HIS POWERFUL SENSE OF SMELL LED HIM ALONG A TRAIL...

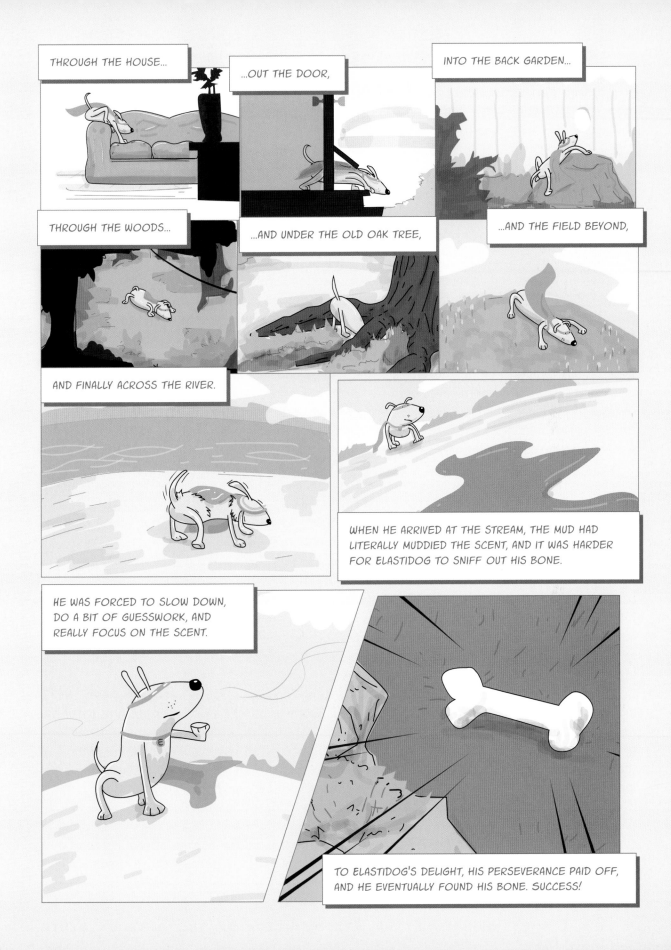

Elastidog's pursuit of his bone is kind of like the nervous system. There are pathways between the brain and the soft tissues (skin, fascia, muscles, tendons, and ligaments) that carry signals so your brain understands what's happening in your tissues and your tissues get the indication to move. Every function in the body begins in the brain and is carried out through the transmission of impulses.[17]

INTERESTING FACT: These pathways occur not just through the neural pathways but also through the bloodstream, lymphatic system, cerebrospinal fluid, and what are called "ground substances"—basically watery, gooey stuff between all the other organs.[18]

One of the ways in which hypermobility affects a person is that the signals between the brain and the soft tissues end up muddied, much like Elastidog's scent trail.[19]

We know that joint hypermobility is caused by a disruption in collagen, the body's most abundant protein that makes up the soft tissues, including the muscles, blood vessels, and skin. Due to that disruption, signals don't get to the brain as efficiently or as quickly as they should.[19] Just as Elastidog had to slow down and do some guesswork once the trail got muddy, hypermobile people's nervous systems also get baffled and impeded.[11] Bendy Peeps are often labeled as clumsy or uncoordinated because of this lack of proprioception (hello, random bruises of unknown origin!).[20] And, because we don't know any different—this state is normal and natural for us—we're completely unaware of the disconnect. We are often desensitized to feelings of weakness, pain, and imbalance.

And so we carry on doing things in the way we have always done them.

Imagine that Elastidog's path from the house to the spot where the foxes left his bone could have been a simple one that would have taken just 5 minutes and 500 steps to complete. But because of the mud, one part of that trail got confusing, so Elastidog adds another 2 minutes and 200 steps, going in circles and sometimes treading twice in the same spot. But he figures that because he found his bone, this path is the best way to find it again.

So he hides his bone in the same spot and repeats the same meandering path the next day, complete with circles and redundant footfalls. Day after day, Elastidog returns to his bone following the same path, further entrenching the route in the undergrowth with his footsteps, making that path even easier to tread each time. And all the while, he's unaware that he could save himself a couple of minutes and many steps and get to his bone much more quickly and efficiently by following a more direct route.

This is often what happens with the nervous system. The way we move—and remember, movement can be as expressive as a split leap or as subtle as an inhale—creates patterns in the nervous system. Following patterns that tell precisely which muscle fibers to fire for each portion of a movement is the body's way of making daily actions as effortless as possible. By creating these neurological patterns, the brain frees up energy for other things, such as remembering loads of new facts about hypermobility that you read in a super cool book.[21]

Elastidog's olfactory bone-hunting skills are awe-inspiring, but not exactly a good lesson in preparing for a cold, hard winter when food is scarce. Similarly, the nervous system is beautifully complex, intelligent, and efficient at getting the immediate job done, but not all that concerned with long-term benefits when it creates these neurological patterns, perhaps those needed to lift a heavy box when moving to a new house.[21,22]

A NOTE ON PAIN

Pain is a great way to understand this concept of the nervous system being all about the *here and now* (such a yogi) but being not so good at preparing a long-lasting system for long-term benefits.[14]

Your nervous system will *always* prioritize safety in the moment. When you feel pain, the nervous system often shuts down certain movement patterns to stop what's causing the pain—even if that means creating an imbalance that will lead to injury in the long term.[14,23]

Here's a real-life example:

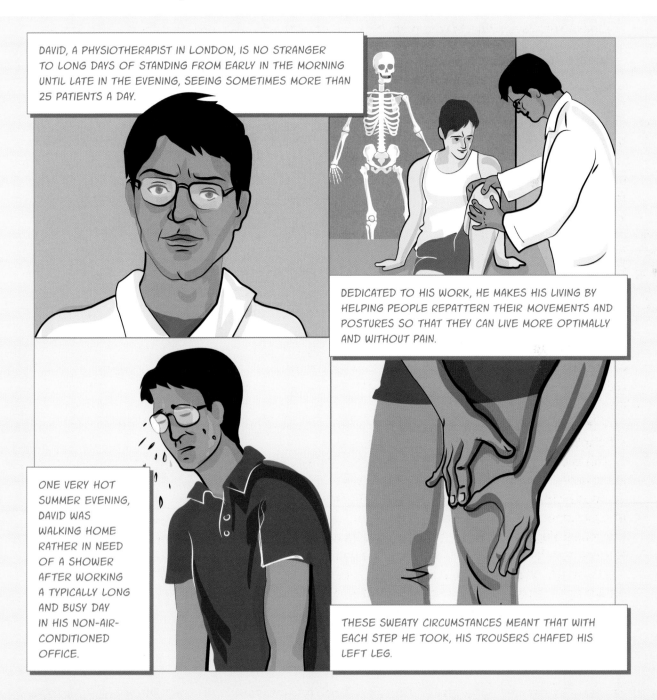

DAVID, A PHYSIOTHERAPIST IN LONDON, IS NO STRANGER TO LONG DAYS OF STANDING FROM EARLY IN THE MORNING UNTIL LATE IN THE EVENING, SEEING SOMETIMES MORE THAN 25 PATIENTS A DAY.

DEDICATED TO HIS WORK, HE MAKES HIS LIVING BY HELPING PEOPLE REPATTERN THEIR MOVEMENTS AND POSTURES SO THAT THEY CAN LIVE MORE OPTIMALLY AND WITHOUT PAIN.

ONE VERY HOT SUMMER EVENING, DAVID WAS WALKING HOME RATHER IN NEED OF A SHOWER AFTER WORKING A TYPICALLY LONG AND BUSY DAY IN HIS NON-AIR-CONDITIONED OFFICE.

THESE SWEATY CIRCUMSTANCES MEANT THAT WITH EACH STEP HE TOOK, HIS TROUSERS CHAFED HIS LEFT LEG.

WHAT STARTED AS DISCOMFORT QUICKLY DEVELOPED INTO PAIN. IN AN EFFORT TO ALLEVIATE THE PAIN, DAVID'S NERVOUS SYSTEM INVOLUNTARILY SWITCHED FROM USING THE POSTERIOR KINETIC CHAIN (THE MUSCLES ALONG THE BACK OF THE BODY) TO PROPEL HIM FORWARD WITH EACH STEP, AS IT OUGHT TO, TO USING THE ANTERIOR CHAIN (THE MUSCLES ALONG THE FRONT OF THE BODY).

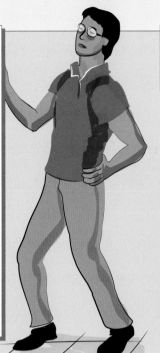

HELPING PEOPLE WALK PROPERLY IS DAVID'S JOB, SO HE QUICKLY SELF-TREATED WITH SOME EXERCISES AND THEN CONTINUED WALKING.

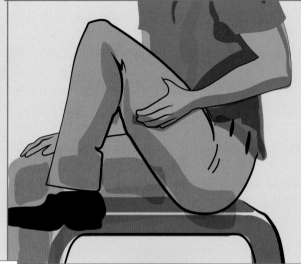

BUT AFTER JUST A COUPLE OF STEPS, THE PAIN FROM HIS CHAFED SKIN ONCE AGAIN CAUSED AN INVOLUNTARY ADJUSTMENT IN HIS MUSCLE ACTIVATION.

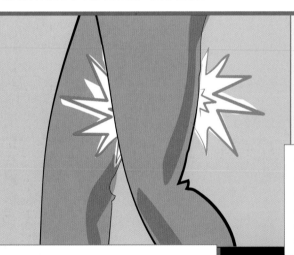

THIS TIME, DAVID WATCHED HIS OWN BODY WITH AMAZEMENT, AWARE THAT ALTHOUGH HE KNEW WHAT HE NEEDED TO DO TO ACTIVATE THE CORRECT MUSCLES, THE PAIN WAS OVERRIDING HIS INTENTIONS AND CAUSING AN INVOLUNTARY SWITCH IN KINETIC CHAIN ACTIVATION.

THIS WAS AN "AHA" MOMENT FOR DAVID.

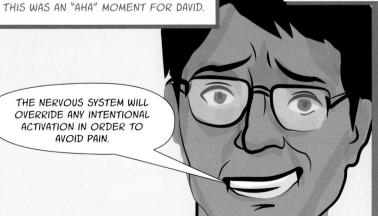

THE NERVOUS SYSTEM WILL OVERRIDE ANY INTENTIONAL ACTIVATION IN ORDER TO AVOID PAIN.

Perhaps you can think of an example of this happening in your own life. A painful cut on your finger stops you from doing a pull-up on the bar, for instance, or a bruised toe makes you wobble in the simplest standing yoga pose.

Your inability to execute these movements might not be due to a lack of strength, proprioception, or muscle activation. It is a strategy that the brain uses to avoid further pain.

As you go through this book, be aware of your body's wonderful drive to avoid acute, immediate injury or anything it interprets as "unsafe."[24]

Considering that Bendy People experience more joint pain and other types of pain than our less-bendy peers, it's worth being vigilant about not pushing through pain or numbing it with painkillers. Rather, get to know the cause of your pain. It's also imperative to learn the difference between the "pain" that comes from working a muscle until it burns with activation—"good" pain—and the pain you feel in your joints after bending too far in a yoga class because you're showing off.[14] Don't worry; by the time you get through this book, you'll be an expert on the most common causes of joint pain and what to do to remedy it!

Finally, remember that pain, weakness, stiffness, dizziness, and nausea are all strategies your brain uses to keep you safe. Anything that causes your brain to feel threatened—such as not eating well, not sleeping enough, hating your job, having a fight with your partner, or bending your knees too far—can make your brain worry about your safety. If you reach its threshold, it might put you in bed with pain (or any of the other symptoms mentioned above) because that's where you are safe. It's not necessarily that there is something physically wrong with your body.

That's why we want you to stay curious about your pain, because often the solution is totally unrelated to the part of your body that is hurting.

ACTIVE AND PASSIVE RANGE OF MOTION: AROM THE PROTECTOR AND HIS NEMESIS, PASSIVE RANGE OF MISERY MAN

Pain is a deep and fascinating subject. Hypermobile people are no strangers to pain, and this book features words associated with pain quite a lot, because pain is something we want to minimize. But of course, pain is like fear, taxes, and that friend who's always brutally honest about your outfit choices—annoying but useful.

Acute pain usually alerts us to something happening in the moment that doesn't feel right, such as rolling over your ankle. *Chronic* pain is pain that is present for long periods, and it may be either obvious or totally unclear why that pain exists.[25] Pain that is seemingly pointless can be mind-blowingly frustrating and problematic.

Every joint in the body has a neutral position in which it has balanced support from ligaments or muscles. When it comes to how far away from its neutral position a joint can move, we have ranges of motion and we have barriers.[26]

Take your hips, for example. Lying on your back on a flat surface with your toes pointing up toward the sky puts your hips in a neutral position. If, from that position, you were to bring one leg as close to your face as you possibly could while keeping your knee straight (feeling that burn in your hip flexors), you would reach a point where, try as you might, you could not lift your leg any higher. This is *active range of motion* (AROM). The first barrier is the point at which you can't use your strength to bring your shin any closer to your face, no matter how much you strain. This is where your active range of motion—your mobility—ends.[26] The muscles and tendons that create hip flexion lack the neurological permission to further contract and lengthen.[27] AROM is known as "the Protector" because this range of motion is safe, and remaining within the AROM prevents injury.[28]

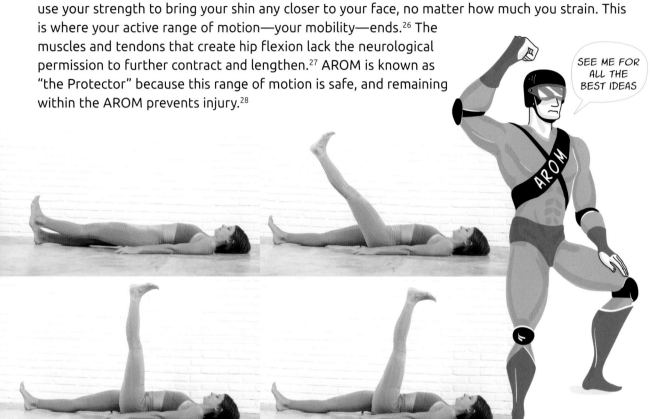

SEE ME FOR ALL THE BEST IDEAS

If someone (say, a well-meaning gymnastics coach who could get a bonus for a gold medal won by the team) then took your foot in their hands and pushed your leg closer to your face, you would be exploring your *passive range of motion* (PROM). That's where Passive Range of Misery Man does his evil deeds on hypermobile people, because it's in this range that all the muscles are turned off and the ligaments are vulnerable.[29]

The general population will reach the next barrier before any section of the leg becomes united with their abdomen or face: the *elastic barrier*. They would probably shout out in pain, "What did my hamstrings ever do to you?!" The elastic barrier is the point to which the tissues of the body (the fascia) and the nervous system will stretch and then happily recoil to their original shape, not entirely happy that you pushed them into a new place but also not injured or stressed by the new ROM. Most people can feel when they hit this elastic barrier, because that's where the brain says, "Okay, that's enough! Stop now!"[30]

The problem with Bendy Peeps is that this signal is often muddied. They don't get the same feeling of "OMG, that's enough stretching; why does this feel so *baaaaad*?" In fact, hypermobile people may feel just the opposite—something like, "Oooh, that stretch feels nice. I bet I can go deeper than anyone else here, giving me a feeling of worthiness that fills the void in my soul."

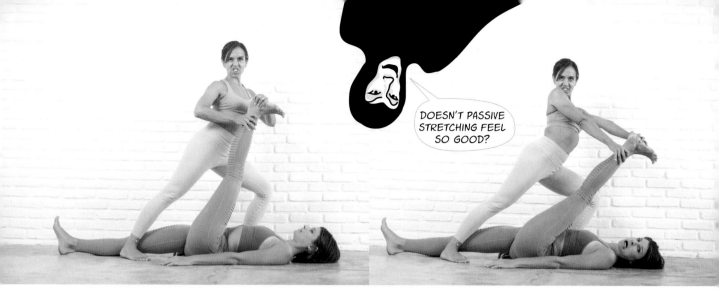

DOESN'T PASSIVE STRETCHING FEEL SO GOOD?

We told you pain was complex! As well as highly subjective. Because while AROM the Protector is a superhero for all bodies, it's mostly hypermobile people who should fear Passive Range of Misery Man and his evil ego-massaging methods.

Most people's nervous systems say, "Don't go any further. That's harmful—STOP!" But hypermobile people just get Misery Man, who whispers his sweet deception: "Go on, you can push a little deeper, and then everyone will look over in awe. Do it! You know you want to."

Beyond the elastic barrier is what's called the *paraphysiologic* space, which is like a little buffer zone that the nervous system has built in.[31] Again, most people won't be able to move themselves into this range because the brain will scream, "Stop!" in the form of pain or discomfort before they get there. Some skilled manual therapists work in this space, but without getting too complex, the nervous system has to be tricked into thinking it's safe or not getting the signal that it's unsafe, which is the case for a lot of hypermobile people.

Beyond the paraphysiologic space lies only one more barrier: the *anatomical barrier*. This is the point at which the body structure—the bones, ligaments, muscles, tendons, and/or fascia—has to be compromised for us to go beyond it. We're talking injury: sprains, strains, fractures, and breaks.[32]

Guess where hypermobile people tend to go to immediately when they stretch? The anatomical barrier. Only the structures in their anatomical barrier don't have collagen organized in a way that provides a robust limit to end-range stretching. Therefore, their joints eventually lose all support and begin to experience wear and tear.[33]

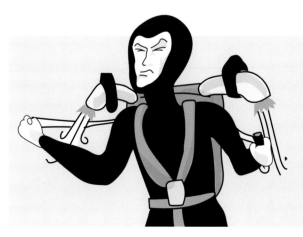

In the following chapters, you will learn how to recognize the active range of motion (AROM) and passive range of motion (PROM) in every movement. AROM is like wearing your seat belt and driving the speed limit in a parking lot. Conversely, PROM is like driving off-road with laser jet packs flaring and no driver's training. You can drive in this uncharted territory, but first, you'll need to learn all there is to know to be safe.

PATTERNS AND HABITS

Given what you've learned so far, we hope you can see that although the nervous system is complex, it's also pretty predictable! The nervous system is all about *creating patterns*. Patterns can also be thought of as habits, because it's through neurological patterning that habits are created.[21]

Earlier in this chapter, you read about how Molly has taught Elastidog that if he sits by her while she eats dinner and waits for her to say, "Twirl, Elastidog, twirl!" then he gets a tasty treat if he spins around in a circle. This came about by creating a neurological pattern. You may be thinking of Pavlov's famous salivating dogs, or perhaps of your own experience of training a dog to do a trick. At first, there's some slobbery frustration as the dog tries to figure out exactly what you want him to do to earn a snack. But before long, the dog learns the predictable pattern and is eager to repeat it over and over to earn more treats.

Every time you do *anything* without consciously thinking through each and every millimeter of the movement, you're relying on neurological patterns.[34,139] There are neurological patterns in place to lift your hand to the corner of this book and flip the page. Even how you breathe is built on a habit that has formed over time. This is why doing something for the first time often feels strange, challenging, and maybe even dizzying. Driving a car, nailing a tricky dance move, and learning to play the banjo are all examples of movement combinations that were probably really difficult at first and required you to focus with all your might on what you were doing, but over time became second nature (assuming you can dance or play the banjo) to the point that you can now perform those movements with your mind on something else.

Habits, as we know, can be good, bad, or neutral. Movement habits are no exception. A walking gait that activates only the anterior kinetic chain is a habit you would want to break and replace with a habit of walking with the posterior kinetic chain activated, too.[35]

That's what this book is for. With the help of the forthcoming chapters, you will learn to recognize when you're moving or holding your body in a "sloppy yet comfy" habitual pattern or posture and to rewire your neurological movement patterns in a way that is optimal.

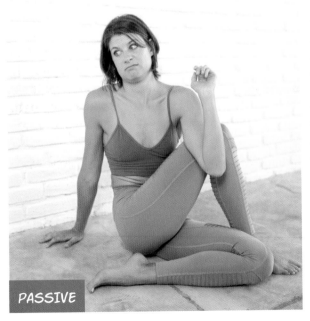

PASSIVE

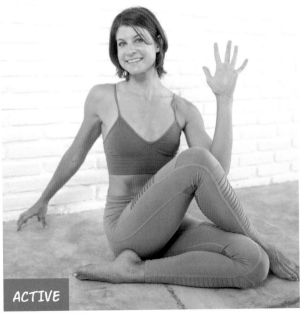

ACTIVE

Be Patient with Your Nervous System

Remember, changing habits and patterns takes time and some perseverance. If Elastidog always twirls to the right but Molly wanted to train him to twirl to the left, she would approach it with patience.

Here's a pop quiz, because we know how much people love quizzes:

1. If Molly taught Elastidog the twirling trick **one year ago**, it will be _____ for her to train him to twirl to the left than if she'd taught him the trick just **one week ago**.

   A. EASIER
   B. EQUALLY HARD
   C. HARDER

2. If Elastidog has performed this trick of twirling once a day **every day**, it will be _____ for Molly to retrain him than if he had performed the trick only **once a month**.

   A. EASIER
   B. EQUALLY HARD
   C. HARDER

3. If Molly has been rewarding Elastidog with the **fattiest, tastiest piece of bacon** every time he performs the twirl, it will be _____ for her to train him to twirl to the left if she uses **raw broccoli** as the reward this time.

   A. EASIER
   B. EQUALLY HARD
   C. HARDER

Whatever you answered, you get a gold star, because honestly, who knows? Not us, because we're not experts on dog training.

The point is, there are several factors that go into how deeply entrenched our neurological patterns are, and there are factors that affect those factors. Let's think once more about Elastidog's scent trail.

Permanent landscape fixtures, such as trees and rivers, will have an effect on where Elastidog walks. These things are like the collagen makeup in a hypermobile body—there to stay, unable to be altered. So our favorite superdog's trail will be slightly affected by these unchanging structures (he can't yet walk through trees or fly over rivers), but otherwise, Elastidog theoretically could walk *anywhere*. However, each time he takes that same path, he feels a little more comfortable with it, and his feet trample the grass a little more. This repeats itself over and over, and that path feels easier and easier to him because the trail widens and becomes worn down, and he likes that it smells familiar.

Neural patterns and movement habits are very similar. Every time you move in a certain way, that movement gets easier because those particular neural pathways are strengthened and any alternative neural pathways are weakened.[36] Bad postural habits, for example, can seem really hard to break at first because you're like Elastidog being asked to go find his bone but romp through tall grass instead of along a nicely trodden path.

It's not just *how long* you've used those patterns, but also *how often* you've used them, along with other factors, like how much your brain enjoys them (that is, deems them useful and safe). So, as you seek to change your habits, please be patient with yourself and apply what's called *progressive overload* to make incremental improvements.[37] (More on that on page 47.)

CHAPTER 2:

HOW YOU MOVE

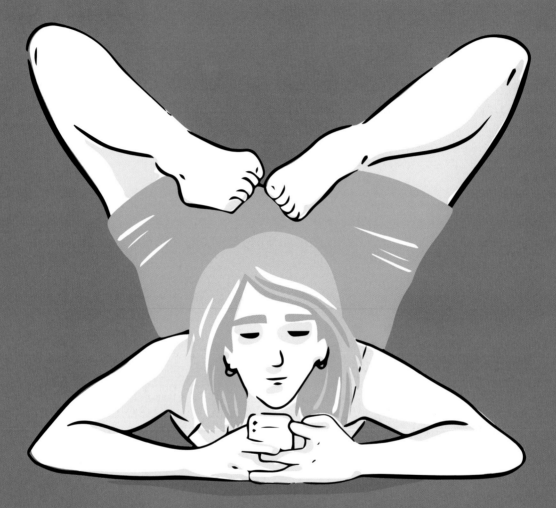

As you read in the introduction to this book, we'd been living in yucky discomfort since we were teenagers, and countless visits to all sorts of body therapists (who made us kiss our savings goodbye) and doctors (who called us hypochondriacs) never seemed to rid us completely of our aches. At long last, we discovered that we were hypermobile, which helped us make sense of all our weird symptoms and empowered us to find solutions, which we've now turned into the tips and tricks presented in this book. Our wish is to see *you* feeling just as awesome. Or, if you work with hypermobile people, we hope that these pages will inspire a unique approach to bring about lasting change.

If the nervous system is the driver of your body, then biomechanics—the science of how you move—is the route that your body takes to get where it is going. Let's dive into how we move as Bendy People.

PASSIVE AND ACTIVE STRUCTURES

Our bodies contain *passive* and *active* structures. (This is different from the active and passive ranges discussed on page 26, but those ranges do affect the structures we will speak about here.) Passive structures are those that you have no control over: no matter how much you try to Jedi mind trick them into joining the party, they're just there doing their passive thing. Active structures, meanwhile, are "your wish is my command" puppets.

Ligaments are a part of the passive structures gang.[38] As you probably already know, these nifty little guys join up with bones at junctions known as joints. Think of them as the sticky tack you used to hang posters of your favorite superheroes in your bedroom when you were thirteen. It did a great job of keeping your poster hugged to the wall if you rolled it into a ball and then squished it flat into a pancake. However, if you pulled the ends of your sticky tack apart until it became long and thin, it did a terrible job of keeping your poster affixed to the wall.

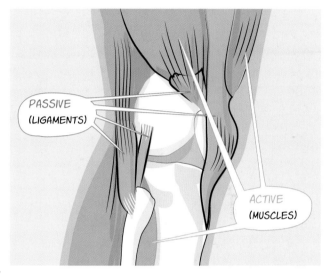

Your ligaments are similar. If you overstretch them, they tend to lose their shape; they don't have the recoil to regain their shape and hold your joints steady. And, because you have no conscious control of these passive structures, they remain soggy and lax, and your joint becomes unstable.[38] As hypermobile people, our collagen protein is muffled, making our ligaments genetically predisposed to laxity. As a result, our poor joints have no clue what a healthy position is, and this is one factor to consider when finding solutions to our unusual aches, pains, and injuries.[21]

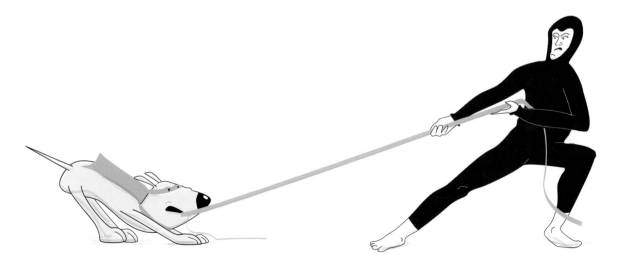

The next line of defense is the muscles, more accurately known as the myofascial system. Muscles are active structures because, like well-trained dogs, they'll do anything in their power to please you and follow your Big Daddy Brain's orders.[39] If you issue a command and performing that task is within your muscles' capabilities, it's going to get done! In fact, with a little persistence and a few brain hacks, you can train your muscles to keep your joints stable even when you're not thinking about it.[8,40] This is the crucial step for anyone with hypermobility; however, getting there (rather annoyingly) requires dedication and commitment. More not-so-good news is that this hard work can't ever stop because your tissues have the genetic predisposition of a couch potato (which is a blessing in disguise, we assure you).

The good news is, if you put in the effort to strengthen your active structures, which activates your brain and improves your neural mapping, then those pesky aches and injuries will be a thing of the past, and you will discover unfathomable superpowers within your hypermobile body.[41] The other cool thing is that once you understand the principles of how your body and brain operate and start applying those principles, they'll soon become habits that you execute unconsciously. Any initial struggle will, without a doubt, fade away until you can't remember any other way of being, doing, and moving.

Before we get into the specifics of those principles in the upcoming chapters, let's jump into the next important feel-good concept— something we like to call the *body map.*

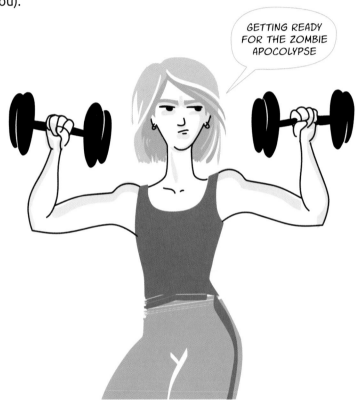

MOBILITY VERSUS STABILITY

To help explain mobility and stability, we would like to introduce you to the man who changed our lives forever: Body Map Man. This incredible dude can change your life, too. Eye him up and down right now!

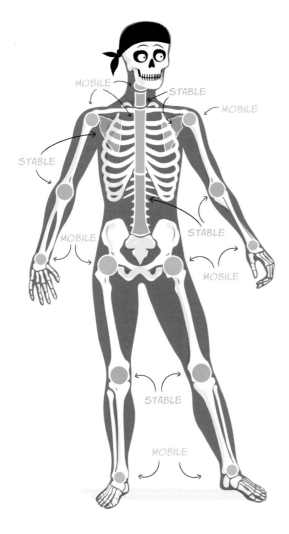

Did you notice that his body follows a predictable pattern of alternating mobility and stability? If our bendy bodies were moving efficiently in functional tasks, our movements would follow this same alternating pattern, and we wouldn't need to keep our physiotherapist on speed dial. The disruption of this pattern is one of the factors that's throwing us off.

First things first, you need to understand what it means to be *mobile and stable.* When we zoom in on individual joints, these two concepts really refer to the same thing: neurological control of the range of motion available.[43] In fact, in high-level athletes, this theory becomes less relevant because their joints have become awesome at both—which is what we all want to happen eventually. As long as you have neurological control of the range of motion present, your body is capable of incredible feats. This theory is useful to keep in mind at the start of your journey as you're doing everyday functional movements; the mobility/stability continuum becomes one way to build awareness of your body.[43,227] (P.S. This is only a theory, which means you should be open to dropping it if it isn't relevant to you.)

Let's use changing a light bulb overhead as an example. If we were following Body Map Man's rules, we would want to keep the neck stable; instead, the mobility (to look up at the light fixture) should come from the upper back. This would help get some much needed mobility into the upper back (thoracic spine). However, you may notice the opposite pattern in the general population. Most of the time, people use their upper neck to look up while the rest of the body doesn't move much. Of course, this wouldn't be an issue if it happened on rare occasion, but if you make it a habit, your upper back will become very stiff as the ligaments in your neck take the strain.[44]

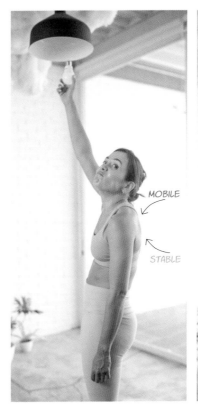
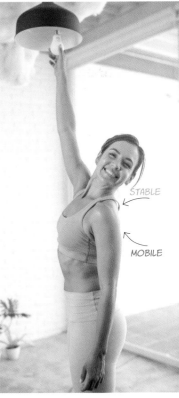

Another example is walking down stairs. Body Map Man suggests that while descending a flight of stairs, the midfoot should be in stable territory while the ankle should be mobile. If the ankle lacks sufficient mobility, the inner foot collapses to help provide additional ROM to help you descend the stairs.[45] This may also affect the knee as it collapses into a valgus position.[46]

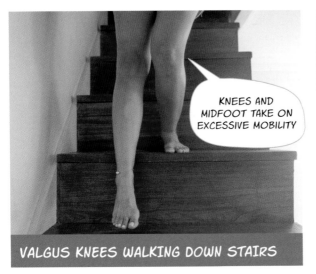

KNEES AND MIDFOOT TAKE ON EXCESSIVE MOBILITY

VALGUS KNEES WALKING DOWN STAIRS

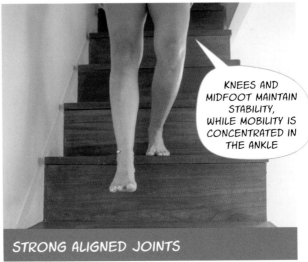

KNEES AND MIDFOOT MAINTAIN STABILITY, WHILE MOBILITY IS CONCENTRATED IN THE ANKLE

STRONG ALIGNED JOINTS

A cool way to think about stability and mobility is to imagine a trampoline. The frame of the trampoline is like the stable joints. It's a solid steel structure that keeps its shape constant. The springs, on the other hand, are akin to our mobile joints; they're needed to make the trampoline bouncy. If everything on the trampoline was stiff, then it wouldn't be worth the space it took up in the yard. Conversely, if everything was springy, the trampoline would be unsafe, and practicing backflips on it would be impossible. Similarly, our bodies need a mixture of stability and mobility to perform safe, creative, structurally sound, and effective movements. You should be able to lift a sofa, go for a run, and tie your shoelaces with your mobile joints giving you the range needed to perform these tasks and your stable joints giving you a strong foundation.[47]

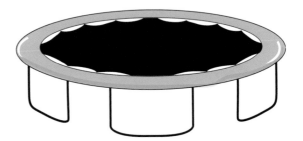

Have another look at Body Map Man as you review this list of the joints in your body that provide stability and mobility:

Spine

Cervical spine (neck)	Stability
Thoracic spine (upper back)	Mobility
Lumbar spine/sacrum (lower back)	Stability

Upper Limb

Scapulothoracic junction (shoulder blade)	Stability
Glenohumeral joint (ball-and-socket joint of the shoulder)	Mobility
Elbow	Stability
Wrist	Mobility
Mid-hand	Stability
Phalanges (fingers)	Mobility

Lower Limb

Hip joint	Mobility
Knee	Stability
Ankle	Mobility
Mid-foot	Stability
Phalanges (toes)	Mobility

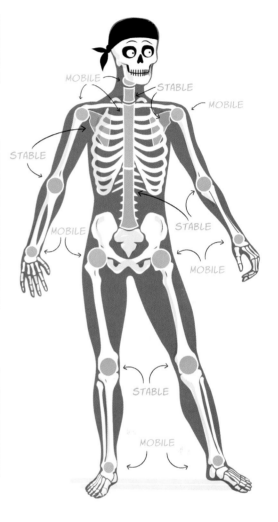

As we move through the book, we will give more examples, but for now, you know the basics. See if you can apply this concept to your favorite type of training.

CHAPTER 3:

THE BRAIN

The single most effective hack to support your bendy body is to start at the top of it all: at the level of Big Daddy Brain, who's ultimately the one that's large and in charge. Although we share a ton of physical strategies to turn you into a superhuman, please be aware that your brain is in the driver's seat! In addition to modifying how you train and move, you need to adapt how your brain receives information and processes/interprets those inputs. The goal is to empower the outputs your brain chooses.

Brain anatomy might not seem like the most riveting subject in the world, but once you understand a few simple principles, your journey to superhero status will be much shorter.

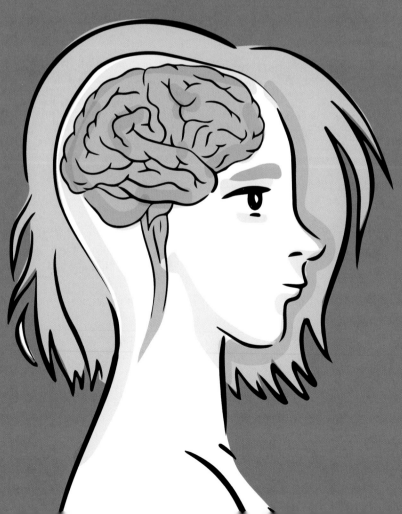

THE BRAIN AND YOUR HYPERMOBILITY

The first thing to understand is that although Big Daddy Brain wants everyone to think it's an OG, deep down, it's actually a very nervous and insecure organ.[49] Its main concern is your safety, and it gets very worried if it can't predict the future.[21] (We have tried to tell the brain that prognostication is impossible, but it just won't listen.) Big Daddy Brain is constantly trying to refine its fortune-teller status by using information that comes from a few different places:

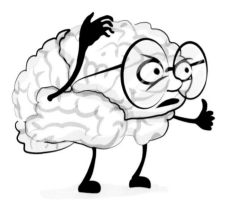

- The visual system (using your eyes and making sense of what you see)

- The vestibular system (your inner ear balance center)

- Proprioception (awareness of the position and movement of your body)

- Exteroceptive awareness (your five senses along with stimuli found outside your body)

- Interoceptive awareness (how you feel: for example, hungry or full, hot or cold)

But these systems only provide the brain with information. What comes next is making sense of that information.[21] And the number one question the brain asks as it tries to do so is, "Is this safe?"

If the answer is *possibly, maybe, perhaps, conceivably,* or, of course, *no,* then the brain produces a symptom or output to help keep you safe.[50] This might come in the very unpleasant form of pain, fatigue, gastrointestinal issues, or anxiety. Sound familiar? Therefore, the first thing you need to understand is that your bendy body might be sending information that is hard for your brain to read, making its nervous disposition a tad worse.[19]

High Sensitivity

We weren't joking when we said Bendy People are special. On the surface, they seem like normal people who live average lives, but when brain scans are done on these stretchy superheroes, researchers have found that they have larger amygdalae than their non-bendy peers.[7]

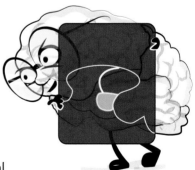

The amygdala is the part of your brain that stamps either a happy face or a sad face on incoming information. It's the emotional processing part of your brain, and it pays special attention to what's scary.[51] What researchers are seeing is that many hypermobile people tend to be more sensitive in general.[7] Hypermobile people demonstrate their spidey senses through heightened sensitivity to light, sound, and touch; it's also common for them to experience more emotional reactivity.[52]

The Vestibular System

The vestibular system is your inner ear. The nifty little contraptions in your inner ear have many important talents, but here are a few things we think everyone should know about the vestibular system:

- It helps keep you upright against gravity and assists your balance.

- It assists in reflexively stabilizing your posture, especially if you get knocked by accident.

- It gives your brain information about the position you're in and the direction in which you're moving.[53]

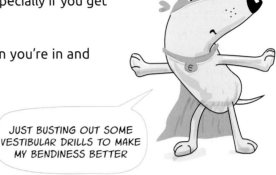

> JUST BUSTING OUT SOME VESTIBULAR DRILLS TO MAKE MY BENDINESS BETTER

In hypermobile people, the vestibular system is often compromised.[55] The result may be challenges with postural stability and balance deficits. If you're the king or queen of clumsy, it might be worth getting your vestibular system checked out.[52]

The Cerebellum

The cerebellum is the part of your brain that's right in the back of your head. It's so fabulous that it's been dubbed "the mini brain." It helps with midline stability and makes you look cool as a cucumber when you need to do complicated movements, such as tying your shoelaces. It is also responsible for movement accuracy, balance, and coordination.[54,148]

The cerebellum is always chatting with the vestibular system. These areas work together to help control muscle tone around joints and provide stability. Consequently, it's not uncommon to observe deficits in the cerebellum in people who experience vestibular issues.[55,56]

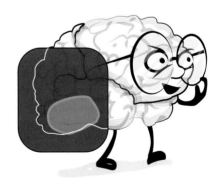

The cerebellum is also in charge of monitoring movements of the body and detecting problems when our joints are outside the safe range of motion—an awareness that is often lacking in hypermobile people.[57,58] As you would suspect, then, cerebellar issues often go hand in hand with hypermobility.[59]

The Brain Stem

The brain stem is the ancient part of Big Daddy Brain. It's been around the longest and deals with all the things that you never think about but that keep you alive, such as your heart beating and your lungs breathing.[60] Researchers have identified that our joint hypermobility family frequently report symptoms that may be related to brain stem issues, such as palpitations, light-headedness and dizziness, vertigo, and problems related to blood pressure.[61] These symptoms are defined as high sympathetic tone, meaning that our bodies are primed for fight or flight even while we are watching Netflix.[62]

The brain stem also has the important job of inhibiting pain.[63] This characteristic of the brain stem is useful for those of us from Planet Flexy because we often struggle with random, inexplicable musculoskeletal pain.

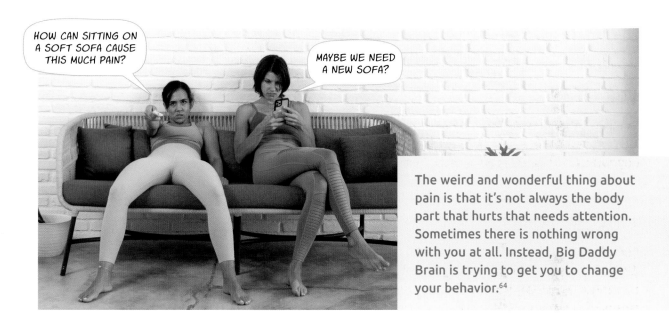

The weird and wonderful thing about pain is that it's not always the body part that hurts that needs attention. Sometimes there is nothing wrong with you at all. Instead, Big Daddy Brain is trying to get you to change your behavior.[64]

Parietal Lobe

The parietal lobe is at the top of your head. It's responsible for processing sensory information. (For example, if you stroke your left arm, you're stimulating your right parietal lobe.) The bottom part of the parietal lobe, where it joins to the temporal lobe on the side of your head, is specifically responsible for integrating multiple sensations, and it's here that we see poor mapping in our Bendy Crew.[65]

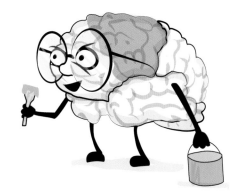

This dodgy wiring means that hypermobile people often gravitate toward movement disciplines that require them to focus on themselves and nothing else. For example, Adell always leaves the surfboard on the beach and heads out for a swim in the sea instead. Celest always loved to dance, but when she was asked to dance with a partner, she promptly tried to lead and frequently landed on her partner's toes.[66]

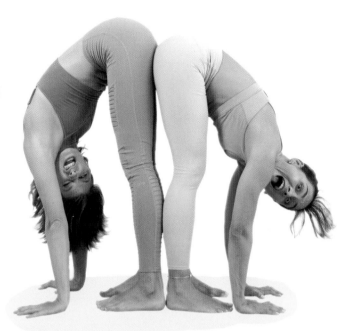

The Homunculus

The homonculus is the "map" of you that lives inside Big Daddy Brain. If we took this map of nerves and drew it to scale in human form, it would look like a character from *Lord of the Rings*. It would have massive hands and lips and biggish feet but a teeny tiny body.

There are actually two of these strange-looking "beings" in your brain. One is the motor homunculus, which maps the movements you perform, and the other is the sensory homunculus, which maps the sensations felt by your body. The motor homunculus sends the messages; the sensory homunculus receives the messages.

In our Bendy Family, these "maps" are sometimes fuzzy. When something isn't used for a while, the brain redirects its neural tissue to what will be more useful. In this instance, our bodies love to flop in their preferred patterns over and over, so the full complexity of the maps aren't expressed and therefore don't fully develop. The more you use the full spectrum of what your body can do, the higher the resolution of the maps will be.

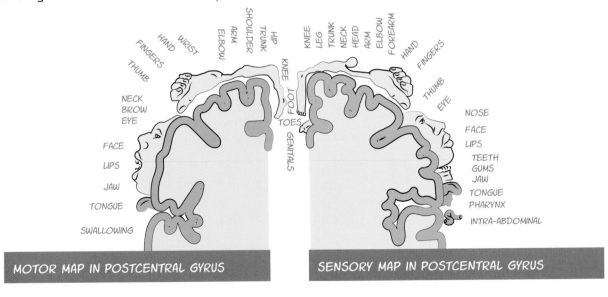

MOTOR MAP IN POSTCENTRAL GYRUS

SENSORY MAP IN POSTCENTRAL GYRUS

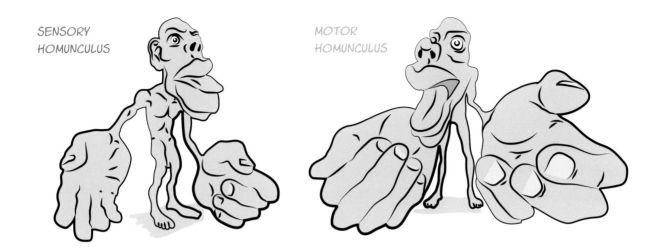

SENSORY HOMUNCULUS

MOTOR HOMUNCULUS

BRAIN HACKS FOR HYPERMOBILE HEROES

OK, that's enough brain anatomy for now. Now, let's take a look at a few practical solutions to help your bendy body and its unique Big Daddy Brain become even more super than they already are.

Mindfulness

Earlier, we mentioned that a person with hypermobility has a larger-than-usual amygdala. This is the area of the brain that processes emotions and can make us hypersensitive to external stimuli. It's speculated that this is perhaps the reason hypermobile people are drawn to yoga—the practice offers an opportunity to be mindful *and* get a workout, killing two birds with one stone. Numerous studies have demonstrated that mindfulness is an effective amygdala-calming strategy, and in experienced meditators, we see a reduction in its size.[67,69,70,71]

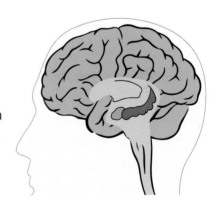

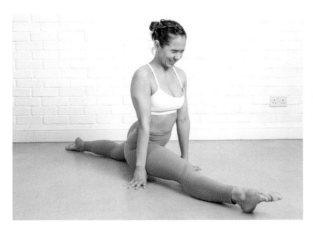

Now, before you go waltzing your way to yoga in the hope that it will shrink your amygdala, our advice is that some people should practice mindfulness *away* from any movement discipline. As you will learn later, hypermobile people have increased interoception (awareness of how our bodies feel), which can get dialed up when we are practicing mindfulness during movement.[68] If we are already overly in tune with physical sensations, making this superpower stronger can be counterproductive.

Our advice is to find a few minutes each day to sit in stillness and breathe slowly. Become aware of your breathing. Whenever your mind wanders, bring it back. If you find that your mind wanders off more often than it stays on your breathing, don't worry. The process of recognizing that you're not focused takes a huge amount of awareness, and even the simple task of bringing your mind back to the breath works on getting your amygdala to chill.[72]

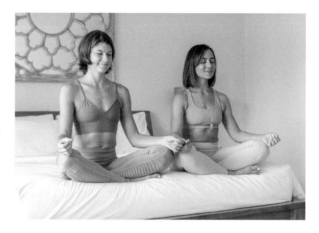

Proprioception

If you Google the term *hypermobility*, you'll probably see the word *proprioception* pop up as well. This is because, in hypermobile people, proprioceptive awareness (where you are in space) is muffled and needs all the help it can get.[20] Remember that if the brain isn't receiving clear information from the body, it gets worried that you might hurt yourself and, as a result, might produce an output, such as pain, to keep you safe.

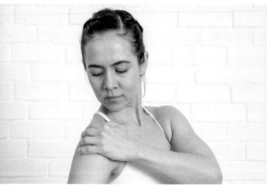

To help your brain establish a clearer picture of what's happening in your body, it can be helpful to provide additional stimulation to the areas from which you are most disconnected. For example, Celest always struggles with her right shoulder, so before she hits the gym, she tapes up the area, stimulates it with ice and heat, or vigorously rubs the area to increase the proprioceptive information going to the brain (known as *afferent signals*). This helps improve the mapping of the right shoulder in her brain and makes her shoulder more stable as she attempts her pull-ups.

Remember that the longer the stimulus lasts, the better. If you're poking your butt in a warrior lunge, you might feel your butt while you're poking, but don't be surprised if your butt turns off as soon as you stop poking.

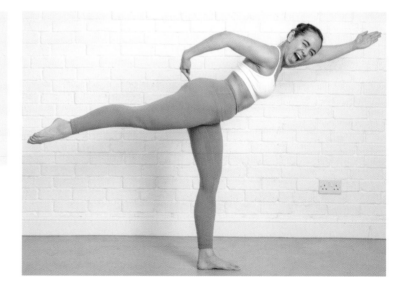

Object Manipulation

Stacking sensation with movement is also helpful for improving mapping in the parietal lobe. The parietal lobe has the job of integrating multiple sensations, which means that it lights up when we have more than one sensory input coming in.[73,74]

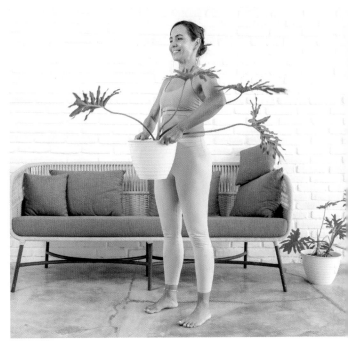

As mentioned earlier, because the parietal lobe has less robust wiring, hypermobile people often gravitate toward exercises that don't require any equipment.[73,75] You often see Bendy People show an obvious bias toward practices requiring only body weight. As soon as we are given an object of some sort, we are clearly out of our comfort zone. But using equipment is extremely helpful in assisting with the mapping of this area.[7] Strength training *with weights* is one of our favorite tools to help our Bendy Friends.[76] That's why something like learning how to drive a car increases your proprioceptive field and develops this part of your brain. Strangely, even learning how to do a task such as juggling enables Big Daddy Brain to integrate sensations more easily, helping it feel safe.[76,77]

High-Tension Movements

What we're about to tell you might make you think we've lost our marbles, but it is actually extremely helpful for hypermobile folks to do their favorite movement disciplines under high tension (that is, to squeeze everything as hard as they can while they're moving).[73] The reason is that it improves the map of the body in the brain (find more on the homunculus brain map on page 40).[78] While we are moving, especially if we are going to the edge of our range of motion, if the brain has a clear map of that new joint range and the nervous system can control the body there, the brain will feel safe, which will improve the quality of its outputs. Ultimately, our biggest task is always to reassure Big Daddy Brain that nothing bad is going to happen, and this tip is another hack for doing just that. Just bear in mind that high-tension movements will zap your energy, so keep these workouts short and sweet so you don't get overtired.

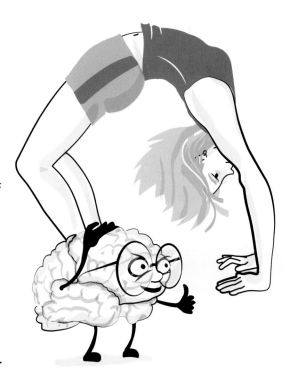

Perturbation

Perturbation basically means disruption of movement. A good example is when you're being nudged by an eager puppy while you're trying to do your yoga practice. When the puppy comes along and perturbs you, your cerebellum kicks in to keep you steady and ensure your movements are accurate and coordinated.[79] It stabilizes the midline of your body by increasing activity in your spinal and core musculature.[42]

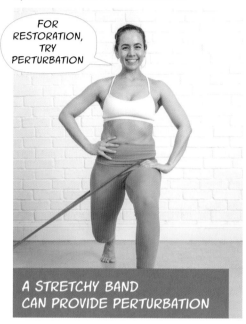

FOR RESTORATION, TRY PERTURBATION

A STRETCHY BAND CAN PROVIDE PERTURBATION

The cerebellum loves perturbation because it has the job of helping you sort out movement "errors" in your peripheral joints. Its other job is to notice and help begin the process of correcting movement and position errors.[79] If the cerebellum doesn't think you're looking as cool as you could, it becomes more active to help rectify the matter.

So, when you add perturbation to any movement, you are turbocharging the cerebellum by making it work harder, which leads to better midline stability and improved peripheral joint coordination.[80]

If you don't have a puppy or friend who can nudge you while you're busting out shapes, a simple hack is to tie a stretchy band around your waist and attach it to a sturdy object. The pull of the band will provide great perturbation, and it'll also force your midline stability systems to wake up.

Visual and Vestibular Drills

Whether you're hitting the gym, your yoga mat, or a Pilates reformer, have a go at adding eye or head movements. As hypermobile people, we tend to keep our heads stacked and our eyes fixed on a single point. Although this can be a useful balance strategy at first, it's also very limiting and doesn't challenge our visual and vestibular systems adequately.[81] Remember, if you don't use it, you lose it.[82]

If you find that adding eye and head movements to your practice makes you feel nauseated or dizzy, regress this practice by standing upright with your feet together and just doing eye movements on their own. Then close your eyes and move your head around. Finally, keep your eyes open but fixed on a single point and just turn your head.[83,84] When you start, a good rule of thumb is to move along the six coordinates of a compass—up and down, side to side, and diagonally.[153]

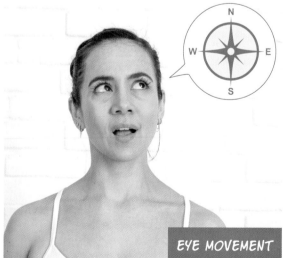

EYE MOVEMENT

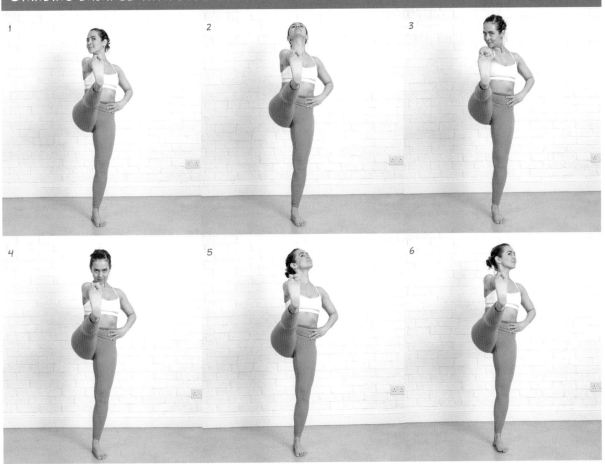

Stability Muscles

A huge portion of this book is dedicated to teaching you about key stability muscles that can help support your flexi frame. But before we show you some of those tools, we need to tell you about how the brain reflexively creates stability—meaning it happens automatically, and you don't have to think about it.[85,149] We're about to get super nerdy, but stick with us, Bendy Genius! Understanding this information will get you to, as Rocky's trainer, Mickey, would say, "eat lightning and crap thunder." In other words, you'll be a badass with a good ass.

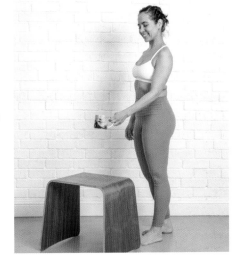

Let's say you want to grab a cup of coffee with your right hand. The right hand in this instance is engaging in voluntary movement. For this to happen, the movement is formulated in the contralateral frontal cortex (the part of your brain on the opposite side to the moving hand).[86] The message is then sent to the hand to get the coffee. At the same time, the ipsilateral (same-side) brain stem sends *tremendous* amounts of *reflexive* stability information to the non-coffee-grabbing side of your body so you don't spill a drop.

When you're doing your training, you can use this principle to increase the activation of your stability muscles.[87] For example, no matter how hard she tries, Celest always feels like the right side of her body is taking a nap in a spa. To help it wake up, she moves her left arm in novel ways while she exercises. Moving her left side stimulates her right cortex and right brain stem. The cortex is taking care of the movement, but her brain stem is flooding her lazy right side with stability signals. The beauty of this is that it is *reflexive*.[151]

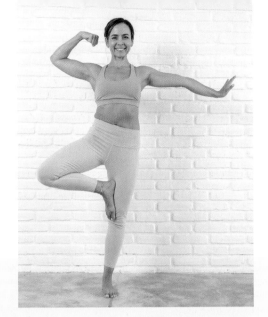

Big Daddy Brain's Feeding Pattern

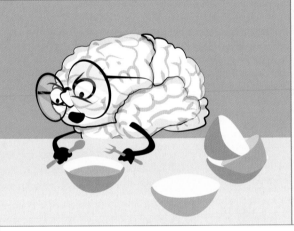

BIG DADDY BRAIN LOVES TO DINE ON GLUCOSE AND OXYGEN. THAT IS WHY A VARIED DIET AND EFFECTIVE BREATHING ARE SO IMPORTANT FOR THE HEALTHY FUNCTION OF OUR BRAINS.

BUT THE WAY THE BRAIN FEEDS IS ALSO SOMETHING WE CAN TAKE ADVANTAGE OF BEFORE WE TRAIN TO MAXIMIZE PERFORMANCE.

BIG DADDY BRAIN LIKES TO SNACK FROM THE BOTTOM TO THE TOP AND THE BACK TO THE FRONT. WHY IS THIS INFORMATION HELPFUL TO US? WELL, THE SENSORY HOMUNCULUS LIES BEHIND THE MOTOR HOMUNCULUS; IF WE START OUR TRAINING SESSIONS BY FIRST RUBBING OUR BODIES DOWN, THIS WILL LIGHT UP THE SENSORY CORTEX.

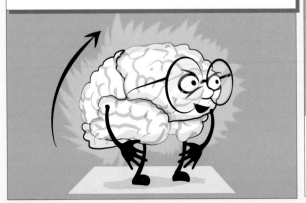

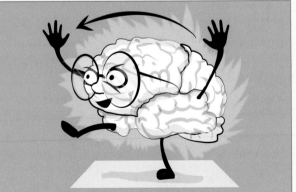

NEURONS THAT WIRE TOGETHER FIRE TOGETHER. ONCE THE SENSORY CORTEX IS FEEDING AND TURNED ON, MORE OF THE MOTOR CORTEX WILL LIGHT UP WHEN IT'S TIME TO MOVE.

Progressive Overload

Think about the different levels of input that we hypothesized Elastidog might have had in the pop quiz about his retraining (refer to page 29). The duration of the training, the frequency of the training, and the tastiness of the treat being offered as a reward might affect how quickly Elastidog relearns his trick. That's progressive overload, and it's another tool you can use to improve mapping.

There are seven key factors to consider: frequency, duration, repetitions, rest time, intensity, tempo, and variety.[37] Let's use squats as an example.

1 **FREQUENCY** is how often you do your squats—twice a day, once a month, or somewhere in between. Obviously, how often you squat determines how quickly you get your well-rounded booty muscles and the adaptations in the butt section of the brain.

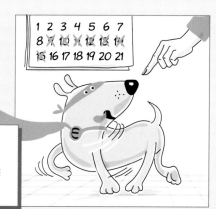

> WITH ELASTIDOG, THE FREQUENCY IS HOW MANY TIMES PER WEEK MOLLY ASKS HIM TO TWIRL. ELASTIDOG WILL LEARN FASTER IF MOLLY TRAINS HIM EVERY DAY THAN IF SHE TRAINS HIM ONLY ONCE PER WEEK.

2 **DURATION** is how long you spend squatting. Maybe you go to the gym and do a dedicated one-hour squat session, or maybe you just do squats while you brush your teeth. The more time you spend squatting, the faster you will develop strength in this glutey-licious skill.

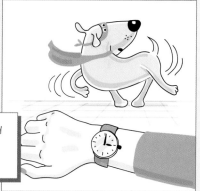

> FOR ELASTIDOG, IT'S HOW LONG MOLLY SPENDS ASKING HIM TO TWIRL EACH TIME. ELASTIDOG WILL LEARN FASTER IF SHE WORKS WITH HIM FOR TEN MINUTES AT A TIME THAN IF SHE SPENDS ONLY ONE MINUTE TRAINING HIM.

3 **REPETITIONS** is how many squats you can do. If you discover you can do only two squats with good form, and your bad habits come back on the third squat—for example, you go knock-kneed and flat-footed—then you need to focus on building up to that third squat. Then build to four, five, and so on.

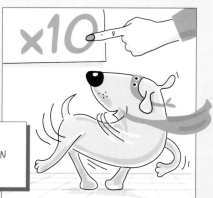

> FOR ELASTIDOG, IT'S HOW MANY TIMES HE DOES THE NEW TRICK. HE WILL LEARN FASTER IF MOLLY HAS HIM DO THE TRICK CORRECTLY TEN TIMES THAN IF SHE REQUIRES HIM TO DO THE TRICK ONLY TWICE.

4 **REST** is how much recovery time you allow yourself before doing squats again. Let's say you do ten squats on Monday, and on Tuesday, you're so sore you can barely walk! Soreness is a sign that you progressively overloaded, putting some healthy stress on your tissues to strengthen them and encourage them to grow.[88] But if you wait a week before doing another ten squats, then you may find that once again, you're super sore the next day. By decreasing the rest time between squatting sessions, you can build up booty stamina. This is why athletes often train despite having sore muscles.

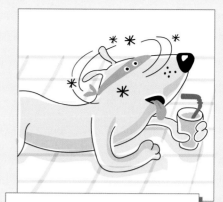

ELASTIDOG NEEDS TO REST BETWEEN TWIRLS, BUT THE LENGTH OF THAT REST TIME CAN AFFECT HOW WELL HE LEARNS TO DO THE TRICK. IF HE'S GETTING TIRED (MORE LIKE DIZZY!) AFTER FIVE TWIRLS AND MOLLY DOESN'T WORK WITH HIM TO INCREASE HIS STAMINA BY ADDING A SIXTH TWIRL, THEN ELASTIDOG WILL PLATEAU AT FIVE TWIRLS AND NEVER IMPROVE HIS TWIRLING ABILITY.

Hypermobile people need to be careful with rest. Yes, decreasing your rest time can be beneficial, but we encourage you to keep in mind that fatigue is a symptom of hypermobility, and sometimes you might need more rest time than other people. How much rest time you need is unique to you. Slightly sore muscles are often a good sign, but general fatigue, like you just don't have any energy to move at all, is a sign that you've pushed yourself too far. Don't be hard on yourself; just make a mental note for next time! It's all part of the process of becoming your own teacher and guru and learning to harness your superpowers.

5 **INTENSITY** is how much effort a movement takes. A great way to increase the intensity of squatting is to add weight. You can also move against resistance by placing a resistance band around your thighs and working hard to press your knees outward as you squat. Once again, pay attention to your form. If 5 kg (about 11 pounds) is too much, start with 2 kg (about 4 pounds) and build up. That's why it's called *progressive*.

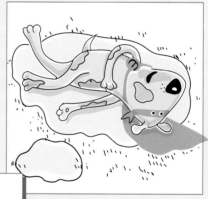

MOLLY WOULD HAVE SOME DIFFICULTY INCREASING THE INTENSITY FOR ELASTIDOG'S TRAINING, BUT IMAGINE THAT ELASTIDOG HAD JUST BEEN PLAYING OUTSIDE ON A RAINY DAY AND HAD GOTTEN COVERED IN MUD. THE MUD WILL WEIGH HIM DOWN, MAKING TWIRLING HARDER THAN IF HE WERE CLEAN AND DRY. THE ADDED WEIGHT CAN MAKE ELASTIDOG STRONGER, RESULTING IN A BETTER TWIRL.

6 **TEMPO** is the speed at which you squat. If you're finding your regular pace too easy, you can either speed up, increasing the number of squats done in a single minute, or go so slowly that you take a whole minute to do a single squat. Either way, the novelty is what the nervous system loves.

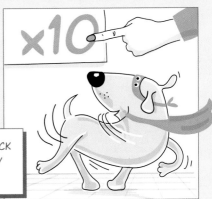

ELASTIDOG OBVIOUSLY CAN PERFORM HIS TWIRLING TRICK EITHER SLOWLY OR QUICKLY. TAPPING INTO THE VARIETY OF BOTH FORCES HIS SKILLS TO DEVELOP FASTER.

7 **VARIETY** is the way you do your squats. We can move in billions of different ways because of the complexity of our joints and tissues, so don't be afraid to change it up! Maybe you do your first ten squats with your feet parallel, followed by toes in, then toes out. Above all, you want to maintain good form by not collapsing into your ligaments. The more varied habitual movement patterns you can create, the more well-rounded you and your bum will be.

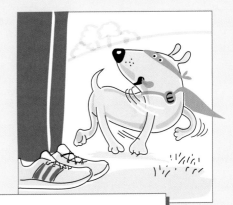

FOR ELASTIDOG, INTRODUCING VARIETY COULD MEAN CHANGING SOME OF THE FACTORS OF HIS TWIRLING TRAINING TO STRENGTHEN HIS UNDERSTANDING OF THE SKILL. FOR EXAMPLE, INSTEAD OF ALWAYS TRAINING HIM TO TWIRL BY THE DINNER TABLE, PERHAPS MOLLY CAN TEACH ELASTIDOG THE SAME SKILL AT THE PARK. THIS WAY, ELASTIDOG KNOWS THAT THE DINNER TABLE IS NOT PART OF THE PATTERN, BUT RATHER THAT THE PATTERN IS TWIRLING AFTER HE HEARS, "TWIRL, ELASTIDOG, TWIRL!"

These are just some of the strategies you can apply when training a new skill, rewriting a habitual movement pattern, or strengthening an area of the body.[89] It's important to remember that you don't necessarily have to do all of these things together! Just be aware that applying even one or two of these forms of progressive overload can help you reach your goals faster.

Please be aware that expressing the full complexity of your amazing brain and its unique needs is beyond the scope of this book. You can head to https://zhealtheducation.com/find-a-trainer/ to locate a practitioner who has an understanding of neuroscience.

CHAPTER 4:

THE DEEP NECK FLEXORS

The neck is home to the stability muscles known as—BOOM! KAPOW!—the superheroes of yesteryear, the Deep Neck Flexors (DNFs). There are two main DNFs, and their secret identities are colli longus and longus capitus.[90]

In the old days, these muscles were epic bad boys, keeping heads perfectly stacked on bodies like nobody's business. However, more recently, the supervillain Sedentary Seductress has glued the eyes of the entire human population to screens. Staring at these objects directly in front of us has changed our way of life dramatically, causing the muscles of our eyes to get lazy. Imagine how much variety our eyes would be exposed to if we spent a lot of time in nature—tracking the flight of birds, watching for predators in the distance, or looking up into trees to pick fruit for our lunch. Doing all this many times throughout the day would sharpen our eyesight. These days, our eye muscles have weakened dramatically. In an effort to see more clearly, we shift our heads forward and tighten our traps, kissing the deep neck flexors' strength goodbye. The devastation is everywhere, and many humans can't figure out why they have achy necks.[91]

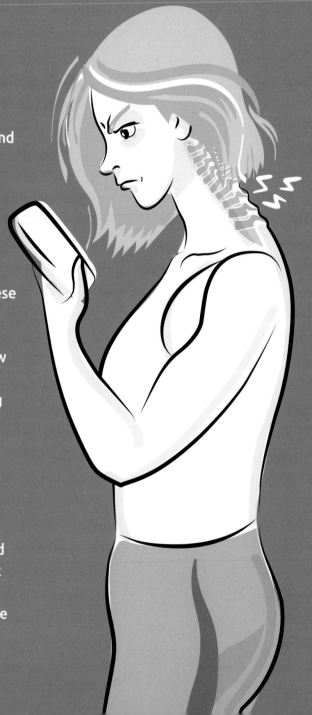

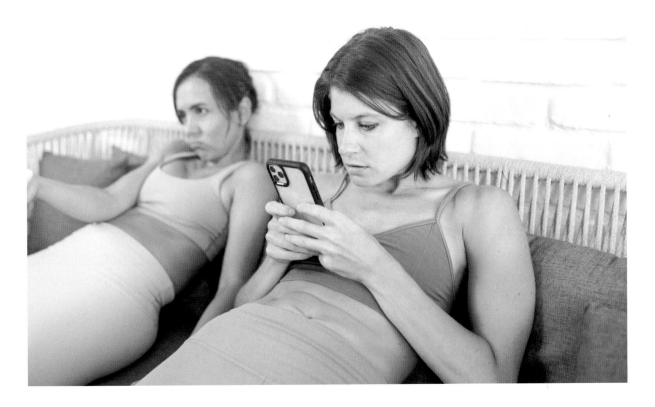

As bodies are fixed in single positions for lengthy periods and necks crane forward, breathing takes a knock. A special nerve—the phrenic nerve—travels through levels C3, C4, and C5 of the cervical vertebrae in your neck. This is the nerve that innervates (connects to) the diaphragm. An easy way to remember this is with the mnemonic "C3, C4, C5 keep the diaphragm alive."[92] When we collapse our cervical spines in a single fixed position and lose the stability to stack the head, this nerve takes a beating. As a result, the diaphragm doesn't operate as efficiently as it should.[93]

In addition to our postural endurance being too weak to sustain a neutral head position and our eyes crying out for a visit to the optician, the fascia (connective tissue) at the back of the neck, where the spine merges into the skull, is likely to become sticky and tight. This can happen to the fascia anywhere in the body when movement is limited. The body is always adapting, and if something is held in a fixed position, the body responds with, "Fellow fascia friends, our human hasn't moved their head for at least a week; this immobility must be needed for survival. Let's become thicker and stronger to help our human out."[94] Of course, what the body doesn't realize is that this adaptation has nothing to do with survival; "tech neck" is merely a default postural position because our vision is failing us.[96] To conquer Sedentary Seductress's plans and help the DNFs regain their powers, you need to strengthen those muscles with progressive overload,[97] exercise your eyes with vision drills, and release the habitual fascial tightness that has been laid down along the back of your neck.[55,97,98,99]

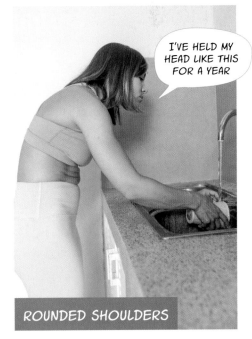

I'VE HELD MY HEAD LIKE THIS FOR A YEAR

ROUNDED SHOULDERS

To love up your deep neck flexors, you can try out the simple exercises in this chapter. They all look ridiculous, so you might want to save them for your at-home workouts, or you can embrace your weirdness and do them at the gym to show the world how cool it is to do neck exercises.

EXERCISE 1: CHICKEN HEAD

The first ridiculous exercise even has a ridiculous name. This one does what it says on the tin: it moves your head forward and backward, just like a chicken. The trick is to keep your head straight; don't look up or down. Stand with your back against a wall and push the back of your head into it until you feel a sexy double chin appear.

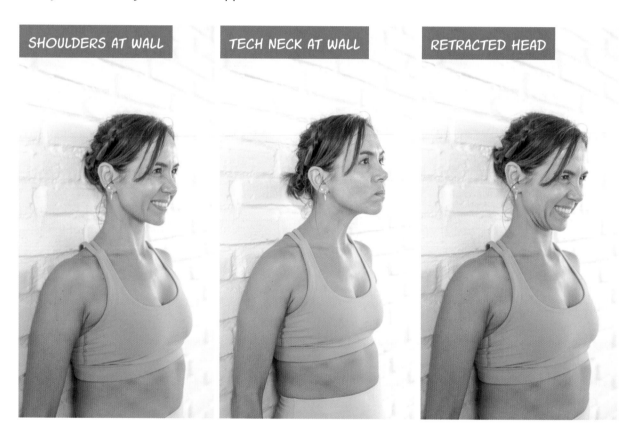

SHOULDERS AT WALL

TECH NECK AT WALL

RETRACTED HEAD

EXERCISE 2: MOBILIZING THE LOWER VERTEBRAE

Once you understand that your neck doesn't have to remain stuck in a single position, we recommend that you up the ante and get creative. The neck has the ability to move in countless ways, but people often move only from the upper cervical vertebrae. Here's an exercise to develop some mobility in the lower vertebrae:

1. Find the joints in your neck with palpation. Take your hand and trace your fingertips down to the base of your neck, where you'll feel a big bump. Just above this bump is a dimple. This bump/dimple combo is where the last two cervical vertebrae live, and it's here that we want you to focus your movement efforts.

2. Practice the chicken head exercise from these lower joints.

3. Try side-to-side neck movements.

4. When you've nailed the side-to-side movements, get your head to travel in a square: forward, side, back, side. Then change directions.

5. Smooth out the corners of this square by moving your head in a circle, still concentrating your efforts on those lower vertebrae.

6. If you want, turn your head from side to side or move your neck up and down. Always imagine the movement coming from the lower vertebrae.

7. Get creative by taking the template from these steps and using it in a variety of head positions. Maybe you can glide your head to the right and do some neck circles over there. Or you can look up and add the chicken head glide. Basically, anything goes as long as you work from the lower vertebrae.

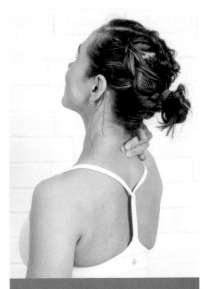

LOWER VERTEBRAE PALPATION

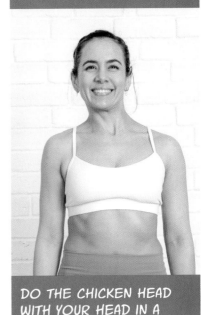

DO THE CHICKEN HEAD WITH YOUR HEAD IN A VARIETY OF POSITIONS

EXERCISE 3: CHICKEN HEAD WITH RESISTANCE BAND

You can apply the principles of progressive overload to developing your deep neck flexors. Perform the steps in the preceding exercise but add some resistance by wrapping a band around the back of your head and holding on to the ends on either side of your head.

Just make sure you don't overdo it. Too much resistance will overdevelop the superficial neck muscles (sternocleidomastoids). A light band is all you need.

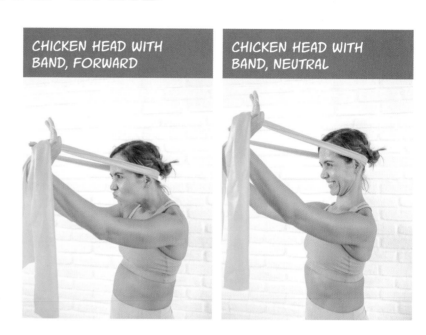

CHICKEN HEAD WITH BAND, FORWARD

CHICKEN HEAD WITH BAND, NEUTRAL

EXERCISE 4: SIDE TILTS

Wrap a stretchy band around the right side of your head and hold the free end with your left hand. Stand tall and tilt your head to the right, then recover back to neutral. Repeat on the other side.

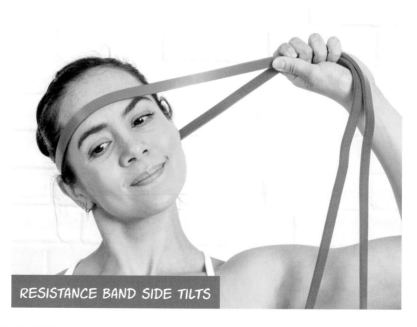

RESISTANCE BAND SIDE TILTS

EXERCISE 5: ROTATIONS

Wrap a stretchy band around the left side of your head and hold the free end with your right hand. Stand tall and turn your head away from your right hand. Repeat on the other side.

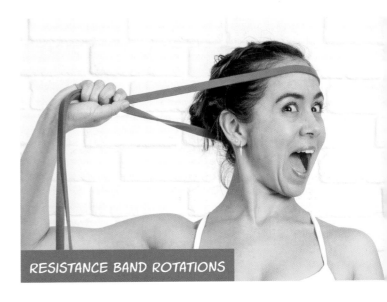

RESISTANCE BAND ROTATIONS

EXERCISE 6: VISION DRILLS

If your neck needs some additional attention, you might be surprised to learn that a trip to the eye doctor may help. You see, you can do all the neck-strengthening exercises in the world, but if you're squinting to see your monitor, you'll go right back to your craned neck position for the rest of the day. But even eye doctors have limitations. Although they do a great job of checking how your eyes are performing in a room while you're sitting still, this isn't what your eyes are doing when you're on the climbing wall, playing soccer, or riding your mountain bike. That's why it's important to strengthen your vision with specialized drills that can improve your vision without the need for glasses or contacts.[100] These drills involve moving your eyes around in various patterns to make the eye muscles stronger. We've also included more specialized drills to practice daily if your eyes need tuning up.

It's beyond the scope of this book to explain the full benefits of vision drills, but take our word for it: vision drills are the BOMB! When you do these drills, you'll be stimulating *soooo* many brain areas and improving not only your vision but also your overall function. In this book, we talk about the brain stem, cerebellum, cortex...all of these and so many more can be improved by adding vision drills to your daily routine.

CAUTION!

If you can get away from glasses, don't use them. If your vision is too blurry while you're doing these exercises without glasses, wear glasses for the first couple of weeks and slowly wean yourself off of them.

Be consistent and do 10 to 20 minutes of vision drills a day, 5 times a week. It's even better if you can spread these sessions throughout the day.

SAFETY FIRST

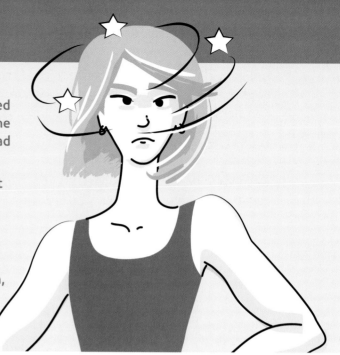

At first, you might want to do these drills while seated so you can make sure you're safe, but once you get the hang of them, use the concept of progressive overload and do the exercises in a variety of body positions.

Be careful not to overdo it. It's common to strain, but straining is counterproductive. Make time between exercises to relax and breathe deeply. Relaxation is often the key to better vision.

If at any time you find yourself getting dizzy, your eyesight goes blurry, or you experience double vision, stop doing these drills and speak to a healthcare provider.

Visual Relaxation Drills

Between visual exercises or long periods in front of a screen, reset and let your eyes relax to prevent straining. An easy way to do so is to look in the distance and relax your gaze for 20 to 30 seconds. You can also blink rapidly for 5 to 10 seconds, which is surprisingly challenging at first.

Also give yourself an eye spa by gently massage your eye sockets:

1. Place three fingers on the bony ridge under your eyes.

2. Place your index fingers around your inner eye area and push up slightly into the ridge of your nose.

3. Place your index fingers on the outer corners of your eyes at the bony ridge.

4. Use your thumbs or three fingers and work on the bony ridge above your eyes.

5. Use your index and middle fingers to press very lightly at the centers of your eyes (only fingertip contact, as if you were powdering a baby's butt).

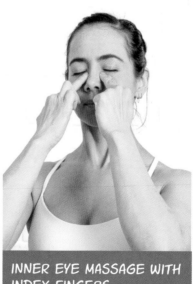

INNER EYE MASSAGE WITH INDEX FINGERS

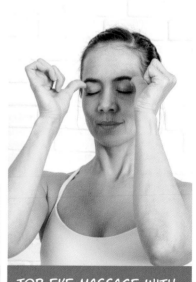

TOP EYE MASSAGE WITH THUMBS

You also can try palming to relaxing your eyes:

1. Cover your eyes like you're going to play hide-and-seek. (Don't push hard.) No peeking! Wait until any flashing light or light seeping through your eyelids stops and you experience pure darkness.

2. Hold for 30 seconds, then relax.

3. Recheck your distance vision. Distance vision requires your eyes to relax.

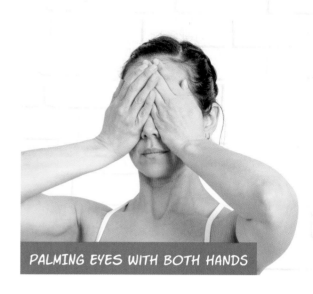

PALMING EYES WITH BOTH HANDS

Baseline Testing to Discover Your Starting Point

You may want to do some baseline tests to find out what your vision is like before you start doing the drills. After a couple of weeks of exercising, you can do these tests again to see how your vision has changed.

Snellen Chart Test

This is the typical eye test where you play peek-a-boo with a chart like you'd find in an eye doctor's office. You can easily order one of these charts online.

1. Hang the chart on a wall and stand 20 feet away from it.

2. Test each eye by cupping it. Your eyes are delicate, so try not to press into your eye and blur your vision.

3. Read only until you can't make out all the letters clearly. Make a note of where it gets tricky. The following drills will improve your vision, so you can check your progress after performing the exercises for some time.

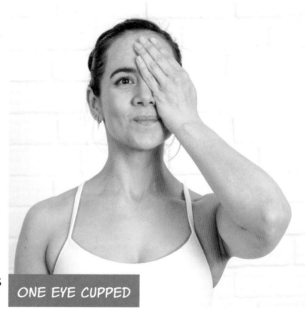

ONE EYE CUPPED

Distance Vision Assessment

Focus on an object at whatever distance you can clearly see. Make a note of the distance and preserve a photographic memory of the object's clarity. As your vision improves, practice observing objects from farther away.

Eye Isometrics

An isometric contraction occurs when a muscle contracts in a fixed position. We have a bunch of fancy muscles for eye movement, and this exercise strengthens them. The goal is to separate the movement of your head from the movement of your eyes. Hold each isometric contraction for 5 seconds.

1. Grab a lollipop (a post–vision drill incentive), pen, or stick. Hold it at arm's length with one hand. Move your hand out to your side (for example, if the object is in your right hand, move your hand to the right). Follow the object with your eyes while keeping your head still. Hold for 5 seconds.

2. Bring the object back to center, switch hands, and smoothly move the object to the other side. Hold for 5 seconds.

3. Try vertical movement by moving your arm upward. Follow the object with your eyes as high as you can and hold for 5 seconds.

4. Move your hand downward as low as your eyes can follow. Hold for 5 seconds.

5. Move the object on the diagonal—upper right, lower right, upper left, and lower left—and follow the object with your eyes. Hold for 5 seconds in each direction.

Try filming yourself so you can see whether both eyes are moving together.

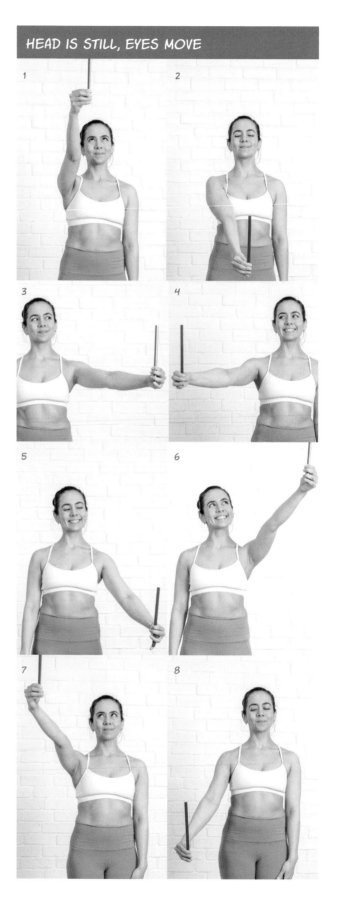

HEAD IS STILL, EYES MOVE

Eye Circles

In this exercise, you focus on the object with your eyes and ignore the instinctive desire to move your head.

1. Hold the lollipop, pen, or stick in one hand and move it in a circle clockwise three times as you follow it with your eyes.

2. Move the object in a circle counterclockwise three times as you follow it with your eyes.

3. After you've done both directions, do a quick scan of your body to determine whether you were tensing up, holding your breath, or straining. If you notice straining, do a circle half the size. If it was easy-peasy, change the distance and draw a bigger circle.

HEAD ROTATES, EYES ARE STILL

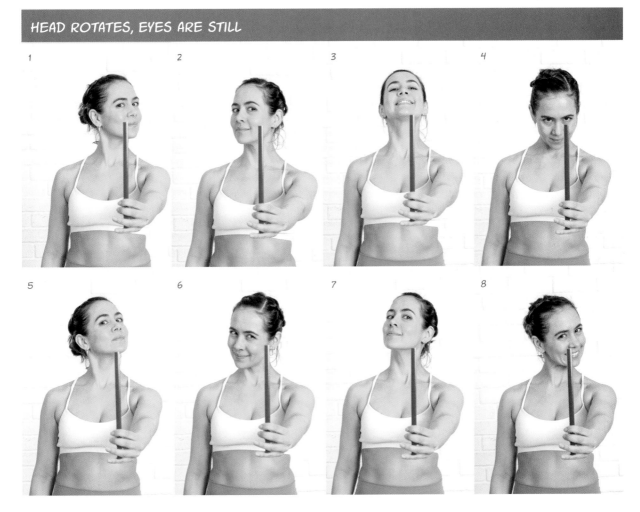

Eye Spirals

The goal with this exercise is to keep your eyes coordinated and focused on an object (for example, a lollipop) as you draw circles with the object.

1. Start with the object at your nose and slowly spiral it away from you, taking 30 seconds to move it away from your nose and 30 seconds to move it back toward your nose. Gradually increase the size of the spiral as it travels away from you and decrease as it comes back toward you.

2. When you're ready for a spicier version, add a dash of progressive overload by changing the size of the spiral and the speed at which you move the object. Move the spiral from low to high and high to low, taking 10 seconds to spiral up and 10 seconds to go back down.

   Before you go on, do a reset by performing the palming exercise on page 57.

EYE SPIRALS

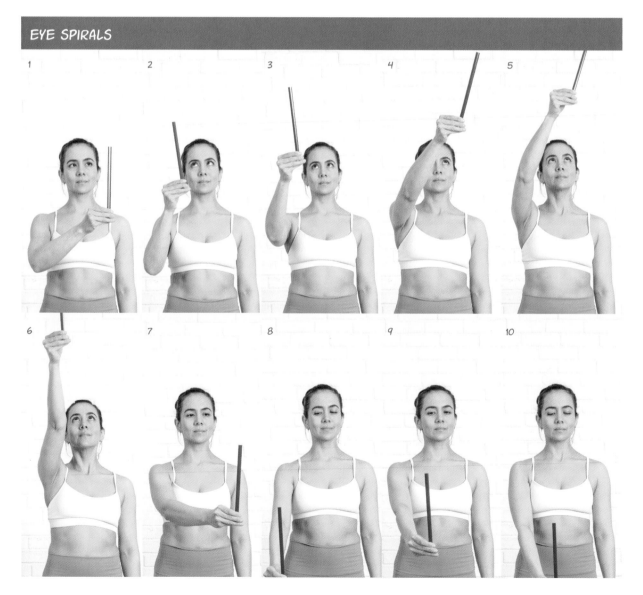

Big H

After giving your eyes a little rest, try this exercise:

1. Hold a lollipop, pen, or stick out in front of you. Move it to one side and let your eyes follow it.

2. Draw a vertical line from the endpoint of the horizontal line to form one side of the letter H.

3. Move the object back to center and perform the same movements on the opposite side.

4. Repeat Steps 1 through 3 two more times.

5. Progressive overload this bad boy by performing the exercise without the object. Just imagine you're moving an object as you move your eyes to draw an H. Tricky, right?

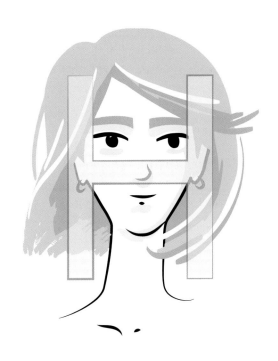

Not so tricky after all? Try writing ABC forward and backward. It's harder to get both sides coordinating.

Lollipop Push-Ups

Ready to rep out some push-ups? You're in luck. This time it's lollipop eye push-ups, which help short-sighted focus and those whose eyes get tired while reading.

Bring a lollipop, pen, or stick really close to your nose and then slowly move it back away from you, following the object with your eyes. Perform 3 to 5 repetitions.

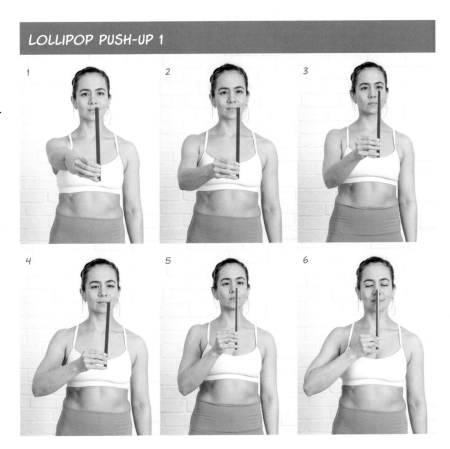

LOLLIPOP PUSH-UP 1

In this version of the lollipop push-up, you work on shifting from close focus to distant focus:

1. Bring the lollipop, pen, or stick to your nose, then lift your eyes and look into the distance.

2. Focus again on the object, move it away from your nose, and then move your eyes off the object to look into the distance again.

3. Focus on the object and repeat the sequence.

LOLLIPOP PUSH-UP 2

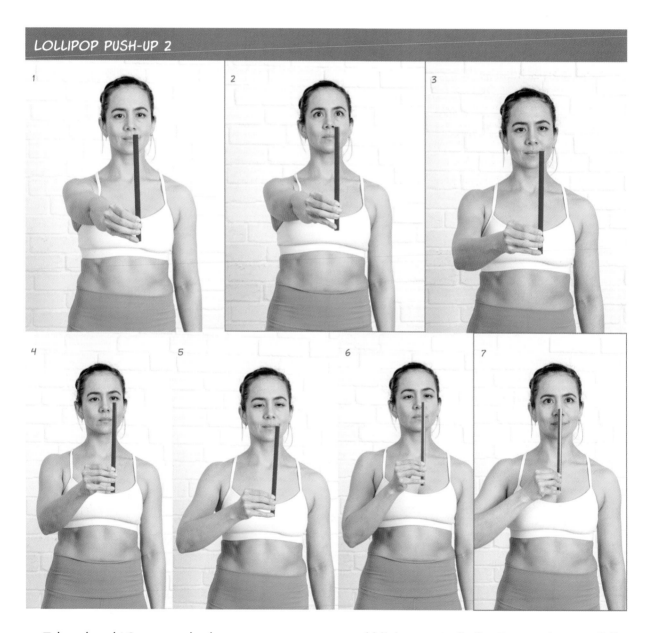

Take a break! Scan your body, massage your eyes, and blink repeatedly for 5 seconds. Hopefully, your eyes are feeling ready to go again.

Eye Switches

This one will get you sweaty! Go for 20 reps in each direction.

1. Hold a lollipop, pen, or stick in each hand and fully extend your arms in front of you.

2. Switch the focus of your eyes from left to right as quickly as possible while keeping your head still.

3. Try going vertically (up and down) as fast as you can.

4. Then go diagonal, up left to down right and up right to down left.

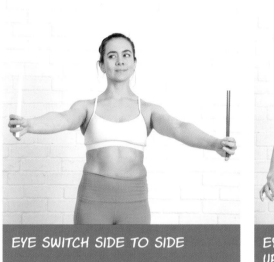

EYE SWITCH SIDE TO SIDE

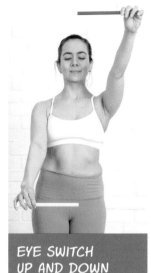

EYE SWITCH UP AND DOWN

Remember, relaxation is the key!

When you're bossing this version, try progressively overloading the drill by increasing the speed, distance, or number of repetitions.

You may be feeling some fatigue in your eyes now. Time to do some palming!

Peripheral Walking

We're taught to be cautious and look down to watch our steps. Instead, find a safe hallway or pathway and take a gentle stroll without looking down. As you walk, gaze far into the distance in front of you.

1. Begin to expand your gaze beyond the scope of your eyes and into the periphery, noticing what's above you, below you, and to the right and left of you.

2. Maintain this awareness and focus as you keep walking.

Aim for 5 minutes of walking, but if that's too much time in the beginning, start with 30 seconds to 1 minute and work your way up.

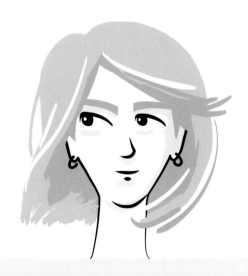

AFTER READING ALL THESE EXERCISES, YOU MIGHT BE THINKING, "WHO'S GOT THE TIME FOR ALL THIS?" THE TRUTH IS, THESE DRILLS SHOULD ONLY TAKE YOU AROUND 15 MINUTES TO DO.

CHAPTER 5:

THE TRANSVERSE ABDOMINIS AND THE PELVIC FLOOR

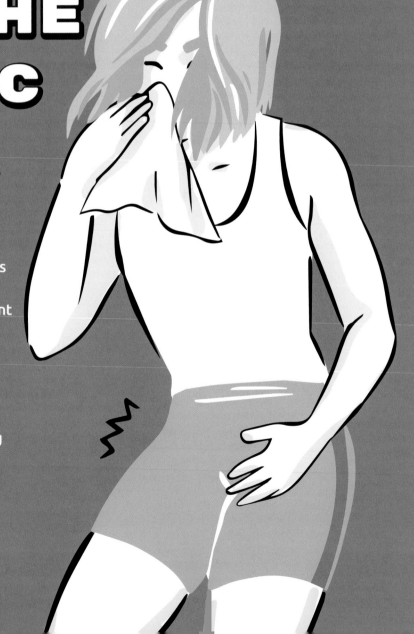

Although the transverse abdominis and the pelvic floor are seemingly separate, they are in a codependent relationship, so we're going to discuss both of them together in this chapter. These two parts of your body are intricately woven together through the myofascial system, and they love tag-teaming on a mighty contraction when a sneeze, cough, or jump comes along.

THE TRANSVERSE ABDOMINIS (TVA)

Trans-Queen Transverse Abdominis should have her own infomercial, complete with well-manicured hands waving slowly in front of an abdomen to showcase its various features. Much like a corset wrapping around the body, the TVA hugs your belly and back, pulling in all your organs and keeping them safe from spilling out and causing a mess.[91,101] The TVA plays a unique role in the body in that it has to know a millisecond before your conscious mind does that you're about to sneeze, cough, laugh, or jump with joy. In that split second, it contracts just the right amount so that the sudden change of pressure in your abdomen doesn't cause any disruption of your organs.[102]

A good example is holding a baby in a wind storm. If you were about to be hit by a smallish hurricane, you'd wrap yourself tightly around that baby—not so tightly as to cause harm but not so gently that the high winds could pull the baby out of your arms. If Sedentary Seductress has had her evil ways with you, however, and you have been sitting for twelve hours a day, seven days a week, the chances of you having enough strength and sensitivity to keep hold of that baby in the hurricane is quite small.[91] Now add the spectrum disorder called hypermobility, and both you and the baby are going to go flying![66,103]

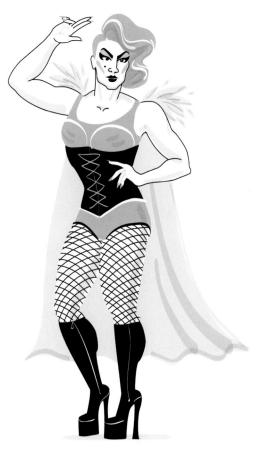

The TVA often becomes deconditioned as Sedentary Seductress hypnotizes you to sit on the sofa for ages, take your car instead of walking, or hop in the elevator instead of carrying your parcels up the stairs.[104] This lack of physical challenge doesn't do your bendy cerebellum any favors, either. The cerebellum assists with stabilizing the midline of the body by increasing activity in the spinal and core musculature, and when you don't move often enough, the cerebellum gets out of practice with this skill.[79] These deficits along with the poor collagen formation in your bendy tissues might leave Trans-Queen TVA struggling to do her intended job of holding your middle in a healthy position.

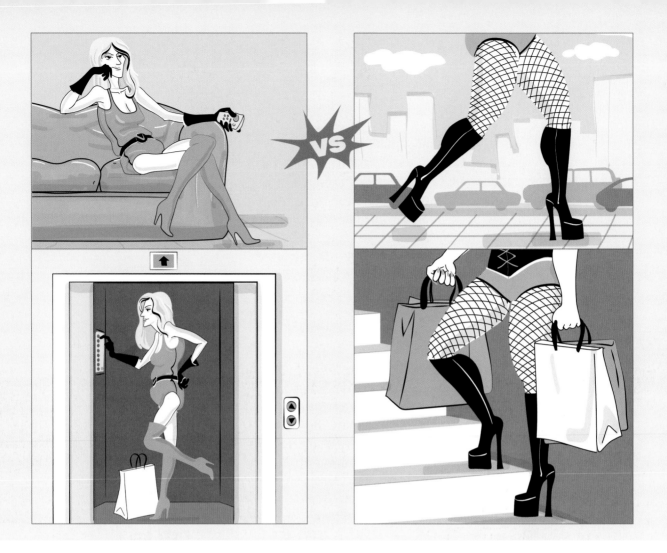

You need to have a stable base to work from. Therefore, getting the TVA, along with the other muscles in your core, back up and running is essential for moving your arms and legs comfortably and safely and providing support for your internal organs.[105]

Think of it like this: when you were little and you wanted to climb a door frame, you pushed your hands and feet against the frame to lift yourself up against gravity. Well, your organs need to push against each other and the TVA to remain suspended in a position in which they can do their jobs. With hypermobility, the organs can't push against the "door frame" (TVA) because it's sometimes too sloppy.

In addition to keeping the organs where they should be, the TVA protects the spine. Not all people with a weak TVA will get back pain, but research has shown that if you suffer from back pain, strengthening the TVA can dramatically improve your symptoms.[91]

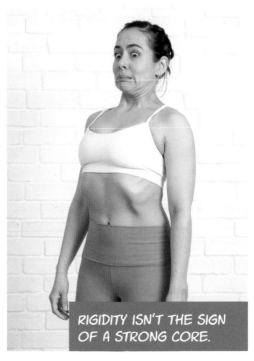

RIGIDITY ISN'T THE SIGN OF A STRONG CORE.

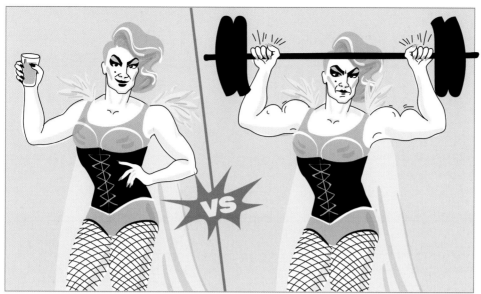

However, it's essential to emphasize that for the TVA to function well, it needs to be *responsive* and *not rigid!*[101] For example, if you were to pick up a crystal glass, your hand would wrap lightly around it with just the right amount of pressure, whereas if you were going to lift a weighted barbell, your hand would contract far more powerfully. Your TVA also needs that level of sensitivity for responding to what it's doing. If you're helping Grandma move her sofa, your TVA had better be working reflexively at the right amount to support your center.[101] However, if you're carrying an empty backpack, far less activation of the TVA is needed.

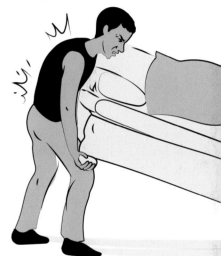

A few well-meaning fitness professionals recognize the value of a strong TVA but in the process tend to over-cue its activation, leading to rigidity. fitness gurus frequently call out commands like "Engage your core," "Grip your core," and "Tighten your core," but these commands don't lead to the TVA strength they desire, because for a muscle to contract, it also needs to *relax!*[106]

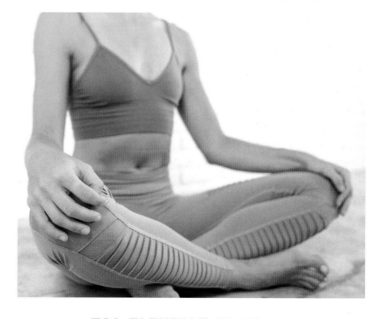

GETTING THE TVA BACK TO SUPERSTARDOM

If you were living out in nature, you'd be lifting heavy loads all day long to ensure your survival. Babies, water, food, shelter-building materials, and firewood would need to be gathered and carried constantly, and these ever-changing loads would cause your body to adapt.

As we mentioned earlier, life these days looks quite different. Not only do we lack movement, but we also lack exposure to varied loads.[107] Our modern-day family seems to fall into one of two TVA camps: in some people, the TVA is sipping cocktails under a palm tree, and in others, it is gripping overzealously.

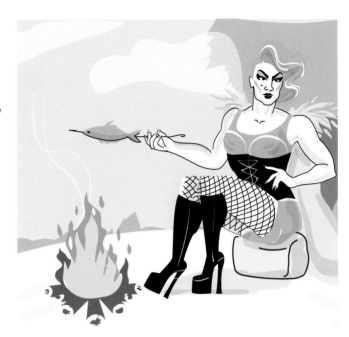

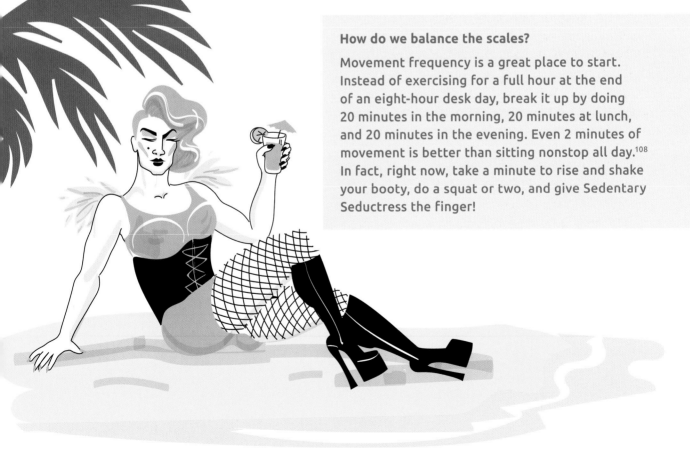

How do we balance the scales?

Movement frequency is a great place to start. Instead of exercising for a full hour at the end of an eight-hour desk day, break it up by doing 20 minutes in the morning, 20 minutes at lunch, and 20 minutes in the evening. Even 2 minutes of movement is better than sitting nonstop all day.[108] In fact, right now, take a minute to rise and shake your booty, do a squat or two, and give Sedentary Seductress the finger!

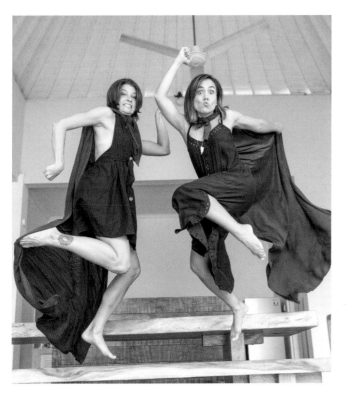

Next, vary the loads and demands on your body by injecting some variety into your movement repertoire. As mentioned earlier, the cerebellum reflexively stabilizes the middle body by increasing activity in the spinal and core musculature.[54,101] You can benefit from this nifty reflexive feature by adding perturbation to any movement. The cerebellum notices "errors" and assists in correcting them, which leads to better midline stability and improved peripheral joint coordination.[109]

The cerebellum also loves novelty. If you've been wanting to learn a new skill, we encourage you to go for it! Dancing, juggling, badminton, or any other endeavor that requires constant progressing is the secret sauce to fireworks in the cerebellum.

You also can work on having a tall spine against load for TVA stimulation—aka resistance training. Research has shown that astronauts are at a greater risk of spine injuries due to the lack of gravitational load on their bodies.[110] The researchers also concluded that the most effective way to make the TVAs of astronauts stronger is by applying axial load. One way to achieve axial load is to step inside a resistance band and perform some basic movements as a warm-up before you do your chosen form of exercise. This strategy mimics the vertical forces gravity would have on your body when you are standing or walking.[91]

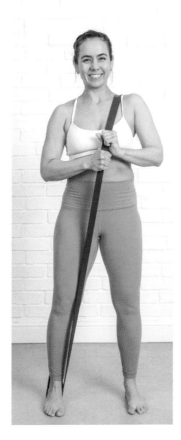
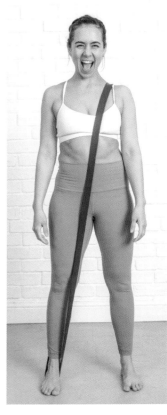

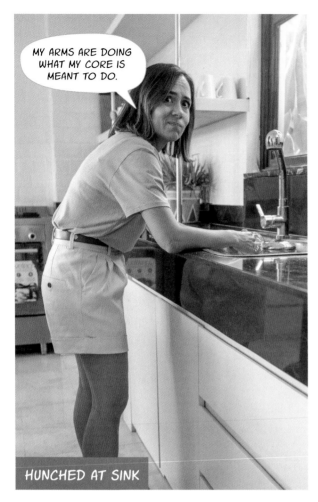

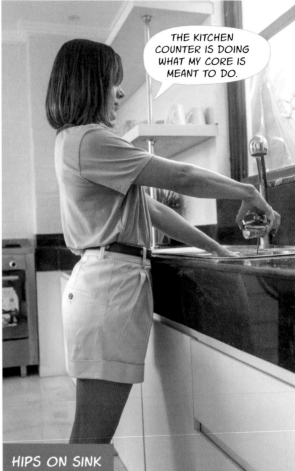

HUNCHED AT SINK

HIPS ON SINK

Vertical forces should not be underestimated, which is why your next TVA-saving task is to become more aware of how often you use external supports like chairs, beds, and sofas, or even how frequently you lean on something instead of standing tall against gravity.[107] For example:

- When you wash the dishes, do you prop your hips against the kitchen counter?

- When you're texting on your phone, do you lean over the kitchen table and use both elbows and arms to just hang out?

- When you're chatting with a friend on the street, do you unconsciously lean against a lamppost or other fixed object?

None of these positions is bad if you do it from time to time, but if you're *always* relying on something to prop you up, you may encounter some of the same challenges that astronauts face when they lack vertical forces.

Finally, you can use your breathing. Ideally, you want to experience a 360-degree expansion of your belly and rib cage as you inhale, while your exhale makes everything get smaller. If your breathing mechanics are doing something different, use your hands for sensory feedback. Put your hands on your belly or ribs and try to feel where your body moves easily as you breathe and where you're stuck. Then use your hands as resistance tools.[111]

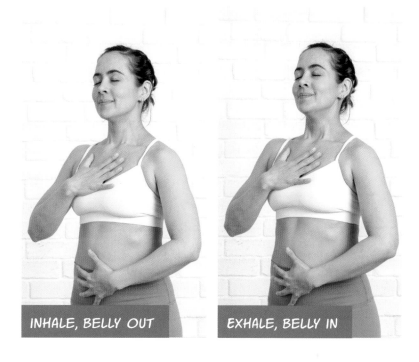

INHALE, BELLY OUT

EXHALE, BELLY IN

For example, if your tummy tends to go in as you inhale, place your hands on your belly and allow it to push your hands away. Or, if there is no movement in your rib cage, consider wrapping an old pair of stretchy leggings around your thorax and breathe into that resistance.

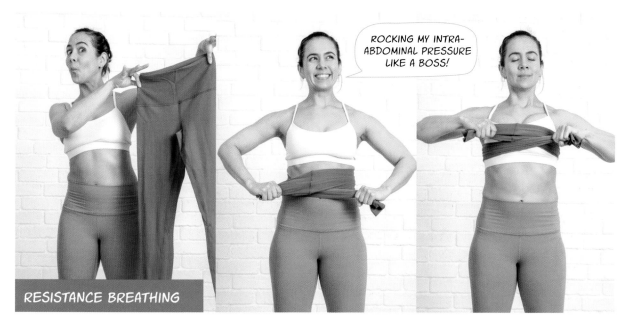

ROCKING MY INTRA-ABDOMINAL PRESSURE LIKE A BOSS!

RESISTANCE BREATHING

As you breathe, your core should not be rigid; it should responsively expand and contract along with your diaphragm.[107,111] (See why we don't want you to grip your belly?)

Still can't figure out what your TVA is and how to feel it? To assess whether your TVA is working, place your hands on the insides of your hip bones where there is soft tissue and try the following "exercises":

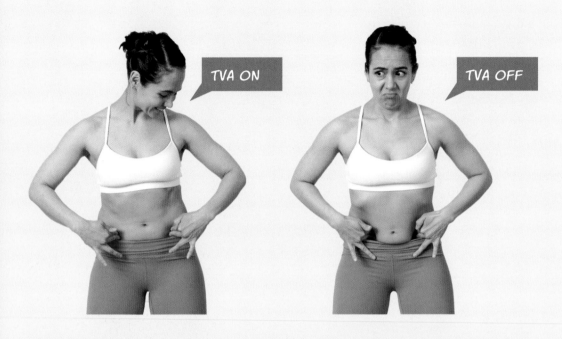

TVA ON

TVA OFF

- **THE EVIL LAUGH:** Deep inside all of us hypermobile people is an evil villain waiting to use our bendy superpowers to take over the world. Because our plans for world domination are frowned upon, we may have to reconsider our strategies if we hope to stay on good terms with the rest of the population. However, one thing we can do without being judged is our evil laugh. An evil laugh—or any laugh, really—automatically ignites Trans-Queen TVA.[112] Place your hands inside your hip bones to palpate a soft belly.[111] Then let your inner villain come out loud and proud in the best evil laugh you can muster. Feel that activation? That's TVA!

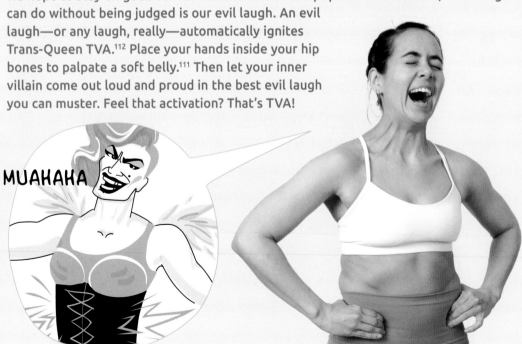

MUAHAHA

- **THE BLACK LUNG COUGH:** Another pressure change activity over which we have conscious control is coughing.[111] In the movie *Zoolander,* the character Eric Zoolander decides that being a male model isn't fulfilling anymore and decides to head to the coal mines where his father and brothers work. After a single day in the mines, he emerges with a cough (a rather soft and pathetic one), which he calls "the black lung." Right now, imagine you have "the black lung" and, as you cough, simultaneously use your hands to palpate the soft tissue inside your hip bones. That contraction you feel is your TVA.[91] (And if you haven't seen *Zoolander,* put this book down immediately and go watch it.)

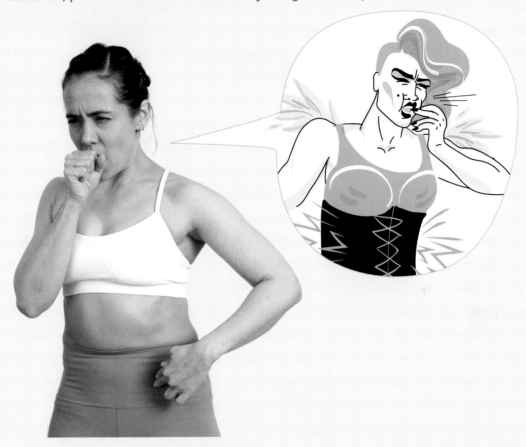

- **PELVIC FLOOR ACTIVATION:** TVA and the pelvic floor share a fascial connection, meaning that if you can engage one, the other kicks in, too.[107,114] We will discuss the pelvic floor (PF) beginning on the next page, but for now, if you know what you're doing, have a go at engaging your PF and feel how it works in conjunction with your TVA. Right now, imagine you need to release a great big fart, and you need to lift up all the bits down there so that nothing sneaks out involuntarily. If you lift up enough, you'll also feel your TVA getting involved.

THE PELVIC FLOOR

Working tirelessly alongside the TVA is the pelvic floor. The pelvic floor is arguably one of the most important superheroes in the body because its job is to support your organs and stop them, along with your poop and pee, from falling out of your body by surprise. It's like a web around the pelvic bowl, neatly but stealthily keeping your organs in place and expertly releasing stool, urine, or gas when it's convenient. Genius!

Secret Agent Pelvic Floor is an extremely intelligent muscle. Just like Trans-Queen TVA, it fires a microsecond before you sneeze, cough, or laugh to provide support for the massive change in intrathoracic pressure.[114] It also keeps everything in place during changes in gravitational forces as you jump on a trampoline. And it saves the day by preventing "accidents" by reflexively engaging without conscious control when you need to lift something heavy.[115]

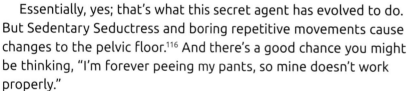

All these examples help illustrate just how crucial Secret Agent PF is to making sure your superpowers aren't disrupted by incontinence. However, it's worth saying that, just like any muscle, *if you don't use it, you lose it!* But how do you "use" your pelvic floor? Isn't the PF supposed to work on its own?

Essentially, yes; that's what this secret agent has evolved to do. But Sedentary Seductress and boring repetitive movements cause changes to the pelvic floor.[116] And there's a good chance you might be thinking, "I'm forever peeing my pants, so mine doesn't work properly."

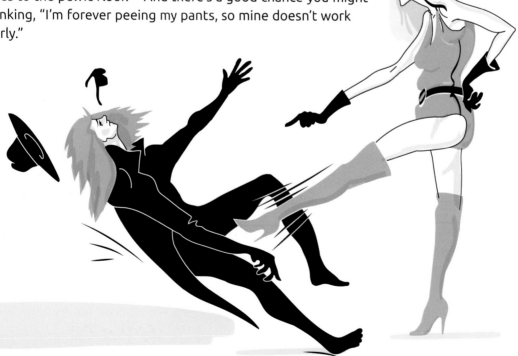

A person struggling with incontinence often resorts to trying to consciously "use" the pelvic floor by doing exercises that strengthen it, such as gripping this muscle for long periods of time. This is not something we advocate, because if you don't relax the pelvic floor, it can become fatigued. This fatigue is common among people in the yoga and fitness communities who practice with the pelvic floor turned on the entire time. Their PFs are often overactive, and they suffer from stress incontinence.[117] Stress incontinence occurs when the muscle has been working so hard that in the event of a sneeze or cough, the muscle is too stressed and fatigued to do its job; then whoopsie!—you have an accident.[106,114] Surprise, surprise.

The other strategy is to do pelvic floor exercises in isolation. Although we think these exercises can be helpful, there's not much benefit to them unless they are linked to your breathing and eventually incorporated with functional movement. It would be like a person who's bedridden getting up to do one squat and then returning to bed for the rest of the day.[118]

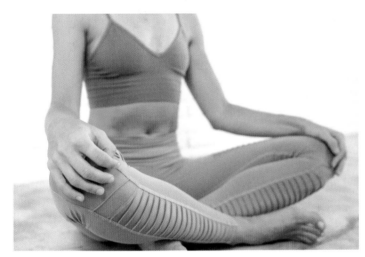

Ultimately, you need to move regularly with a variety of activities *and* do PF-strengthening exercises. As you build up this muscle, you may start to engage your pelvic floor alongside your breathing (see page 76) consciously while doing your favorite form of training. Eventually, you want Secret Agent Pelvic Floor to be firing reflexively so that it's just doing its secret agent thing to keep your organs and body fluids neatly tucked away while you're none the wiser.

Issues When the TVA and PF Are Out of Balance

Because of our stretchy tissues, we need to be mindful of the effects of a sedentary lifestyle. When we sit too much, the PF bows like a hammock, and the contents of the abdomen push down on our PF and make it stretchier and stretchier.[115,119] Therefore, you want to make sure you're moving frequently.

Studies have shown that hypermobile people are prone to prolapse, which occurs when there is a displacement of an organ from its normal position, usually downward, causing it to protrude from your vagina or anus.[115] To help prevent prolapse, be careful not to strain when you're on the toilet. It's important to train your body to relax by breathing deeply and taking your time.

Finally, incontinence is a common dysfunction seen across all ages. We need our poos and pees to exit when we tell them to, *never by accident!*

We know all this is a bit of scaremongering, and these issues don't affect everyone, of course. But they're common enough that we want to make sure you're equipped with the right tools to help your bits stay where they belong.

So you're probably saying, "OK, OK. TELL ME ALREADY: WHAT CAN I DOOOO?!"

Training the Pelvic Floor

To get your pelvic floor working like a boss, you need to activate it with your breathing. As you inhale, the TVA and pelvic floor relax; as you exhale, they engage.[91]

A quick recap of intrathoracic pressure: The increase in pressure means that there is more stuff (air) inside the lungs, so there is more support. With this increase in pressure, your organs push down on your pelvic floor, which is why it needs to relax to make space for the additional air. The exhale reverses this process, which is why you need to engage the pelvic floor.[120]

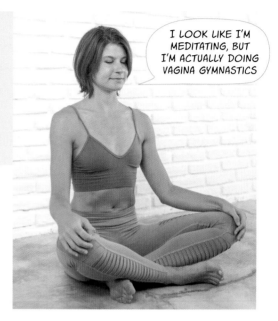

I LOOK LIKE I'M MEDITATING, BUT I'M ACTUALLY DOING VAGINA GYMNASTICS

The PF is often referred to as the second diaphragm.[120] When we think about the way the PF and the diaphragm work, we always think of a dance: as you exhale, the pelvic floor contracts and the diaphragm relaxes. Then, on the inhale, the diaphragm contracts and the pelvic floor relaxes. This dance needs to happen in *all* people, hypermobile or not. But because of our poor proprioception, we Bendies struggle with the coordination. Don't worry; all is not lost. If you practice this dance, your brain will be so happy that it'll start reminding you to do it more and more until it's second nature. Here are the steps to train your brain to do this unconsciously:[91]

1. Begin by breathing into your belly while relaxing the TVA and PF. (If you find relaxing this section of your body difficult, you may want to see a pelvic health physiotherapist.)

2. Exhale with engagement of the PF and TVA. If you're lying down or sitting, this engagement will be gentle. If you are in plank position and your two-year-old climbs on you, it'll be more powerful. Again, you're aiming for a reflexive engagement.

REMEMBER, WE DON'T WANT TO HAVE A STATIC BELLY THAT NEVER MOVES. YOUR ABDOMINAL WALL SHOULD RESPOND TO THE PRESSURE CHANGES CREATED BY BREATHING.

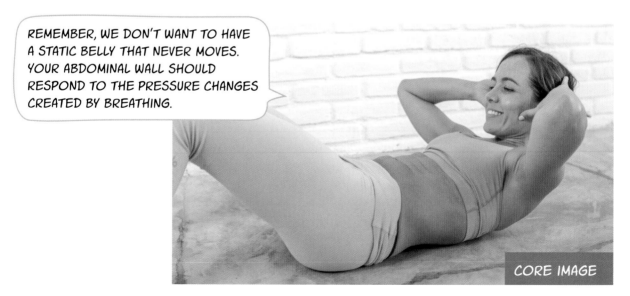

CORE IMAGE

For some people, this engagement is really hard to feel. If you're in that camp, seek help from a pelvic health physiotherapist.

Research has shown that when people think they're engaging their PF, many are actually bearing down (pushing their internals down). This is the opposite of what you want, so you need to be mindful. You want an engaged pelvic floor to feel like you're lifting up (as if you're holding in a poo), and you want this lift to work in conjunction with the exhale.

At first, you might need to use all your powers of concentration to achieve the rhythm of this breathing exercise, but as you get the hang of it, start slotting it into your walks around the park or your gym workouts. As your confidence increases further, you'll find that it becomes second nature.

Superpower-Enhancing Drill: Blow Before You Go

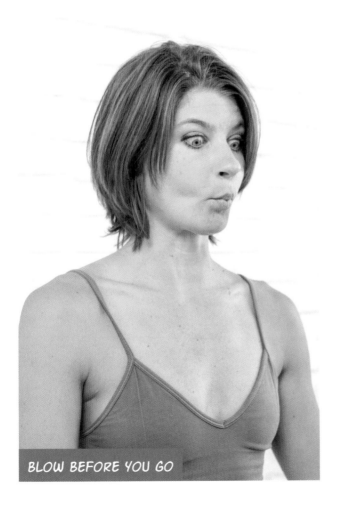

BLOW BEFORE YOU GO

Blow Before You Go is basically a normal inhale that fills your relaxed tummy, followed by then an exhale through pursed lips.[91] (Geeky side note: Pursed-lip breathing increases intrathoracic pressure.)

The pelvic floor and TVA respond to this breathing strategy reflexively, making this exercise particularly helpful if you're very weak.[91] Eventually, once everything is firing normally, you can drop the breathing strategy but keep the coordination between the exhale and the engagement.

CHAPTER 6:

THE POSTERIOR CHAIN

Living out in nature would have put a variety of stresses on and inputs into the bodies of our ancestors, and this variety led to adaptation to ensure the survival of the human species. This same adaptation is happening this very second in every single body on the planet, hypermobile or not.

Our bodies adapt in different ways, partly because our habits and environments differ, so the stresses our bodies are asked to process are unique.[121] These days, however, those differences are becoming less varied as a huge percentage of the population succumbs to the evil mastermind Sedentary Seductress. Modern life has a strong bias toward cushioned chairs, flat surfaces, restrictive footwear, and mechanical devices that move you from point A to point B.[104,122] Some of us who live in bigger cities even have pretty much everything money can buy delivered right to our front doors.

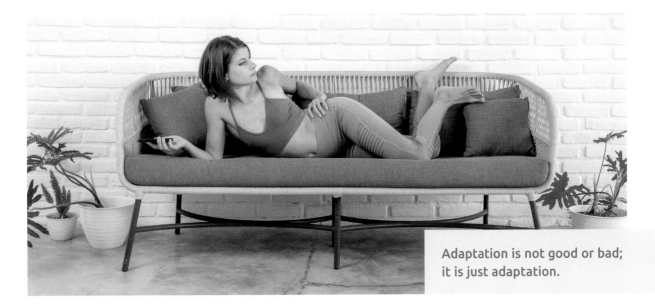

Adaptation is not good or bad; it is just adaptation.

These changes to our environment have been awesome at making us more comfortable in the short term, but they have also removed the stressors we require to live a life off the sofa.[123] We keep saying it, and we will say it again: *if you don't use it, you lose it.*

This brings us to one of the most important physical characteristics the human body had to develop to ensure survival: a strong posterior chain.

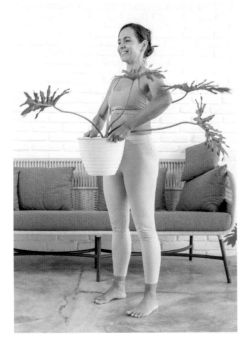

The muscles that make up the posterior chain are the calves, hamstrings, glutes, and back muscles. This chain is strengthened through lifting things (external masses) toward the body.[124] Lifting is a skill that our ancestors would have had to perform regularly to survive in nature. Children would be strapped to bodies, water and food would be carried for miles, and building materials would be lifted a few times a year as old structures weathered and people moved to new locations.[125] These days, the posterior chain has wheels, elevators, cranes, and delivery services giving it an extended holiday in the Bahamas. Our desire for comfort also places our posterior chains in chairs and on toilet seats—objects that have removed the need to squat. With the removal of squatting, so goes the physical adaptation that comes with that action. Sedentary Seductress has used her secret power—convenience—to remove the need for movement, and especially lifting, from almost every part of our modern lives.

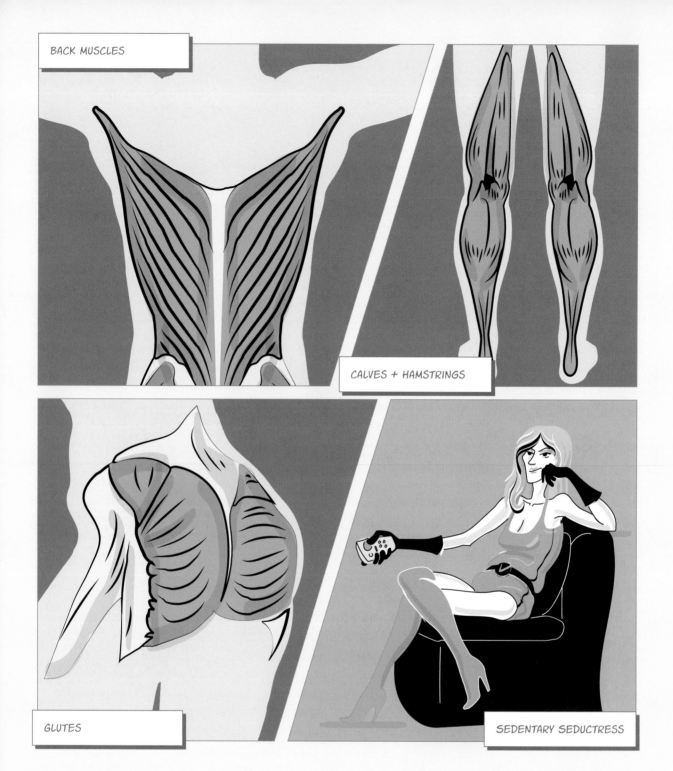

BACK MUSCLES

CALVES + HAMSTRINGS

GLUTES

SEDENTARY SEDUCTRESS

Now, you might be thinking, "Hang on, darlings; for the most part, we don't need to worry about survival anymore. Since we have that covered, can't we let our posterior chain off the hook and go back to living in the matrix?"

We highly encourage you to take the red pill and keep reading...

Introducing Team Gluteus, the saviors of victims of silly injuries that are perfectly avoidable. The team is made up of three superheroes:

GLUTEUS MAXIMUS AURELIUS, our favorite openly gay gladiator and massive fan of the TV show *Friends*. Glute Max is responsible for hip extension and hip external rotation. In daily life, you need his glory especially when standing, lifting, and walking.

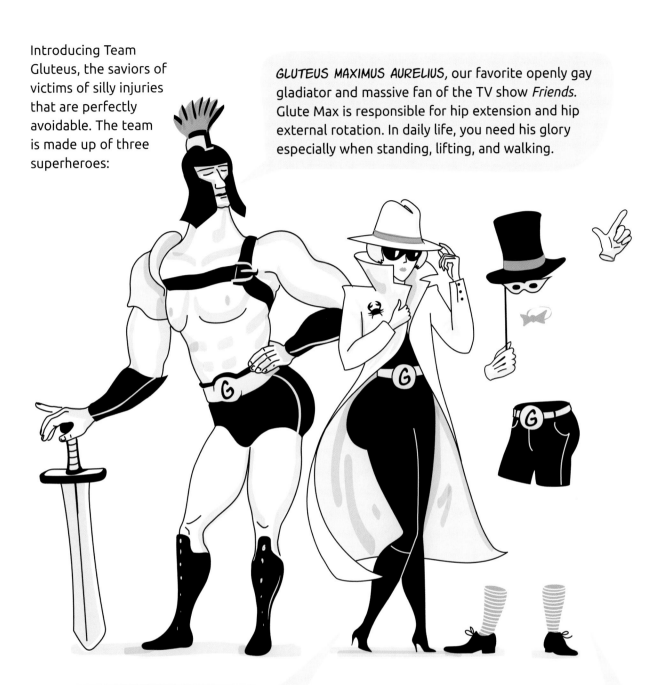

SASSY STABILITY AGENT GLUTEUS MEDIUS, a petite badass whose favorite animal is the crab. We sometimes call her Agent M for short. Gluteus Medius and Gluteus Minimus are needed for pelvic stability, especially for standing on one leg. They also help the knees stay stable.

PHANTOM GLUTEUS MINIMUS, who supports Sassy Stability Agent Gluteus Medius as an invisible badass sidekick.[124]

Perhaps our survival isn't dependent on being able to lift anymore, but our physical health very much is.

WAKING UP THE POSTERIOR CHAIN REFLEXIVELY

Although we are big fans of targeted glute activation drills, it's important for us to keep reminding you that these drills are just one tool to kick Sedentary Seductress's derriere! Some people do butt exercises till they are blue in the face and pink in their cheeks (get it?), yet they still can't get their glutes to turn on.

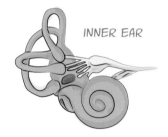

INNER EAR

In this instance, it's worth targeting the higher-order systems in the Big Daddy Brain—specifically the cerebellum and vestibular system. These two brain regions are in constant communication with each other and are in charge of getting the posterior chain to kick in, turning you into a badass with a good ass (and great posture, too).[126,127] In particular, we are going to show you how to wake up the vestibulospinal tract (inner ear and spinal cord tract), which helps stabilize posture reflexively.

Turning On the Vestibulospinal Tract

To turn on your vestibulospinal tract, give this exercise a try:[128]

1. Stand with your feet together and your eyes closed.

2. Do a sharp head movement and then hold it there for 5 to 10 seconds. The head positions are

   – Rotation, left and right

   – Side flexion, left and right

   – Head up and down

You can up the ante by doing these drills while you're standing on one leg. Or you can add perturbation by looping a stretchy band around a fixed point and stepping inside it.

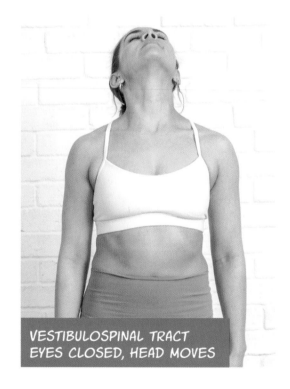

VESTIBULOSPINAL TRACT
EYES CLOSED, HEAD MOVES

Stimulating the Cerebellum

We've discussed progressive overload a couple of times and explained how you can use it to get your body to adapt quicker. Well, it's also useful when activating the cerebellum, especially when utilizing speed variability, doing movements under load, or expressing your full range of motion actively.[129] This is good for the whole body, but to fire up the cerebellum quickly, use the following exercises to work on joint-rich areas such as the hands, feet, and thoracic spine.[130]

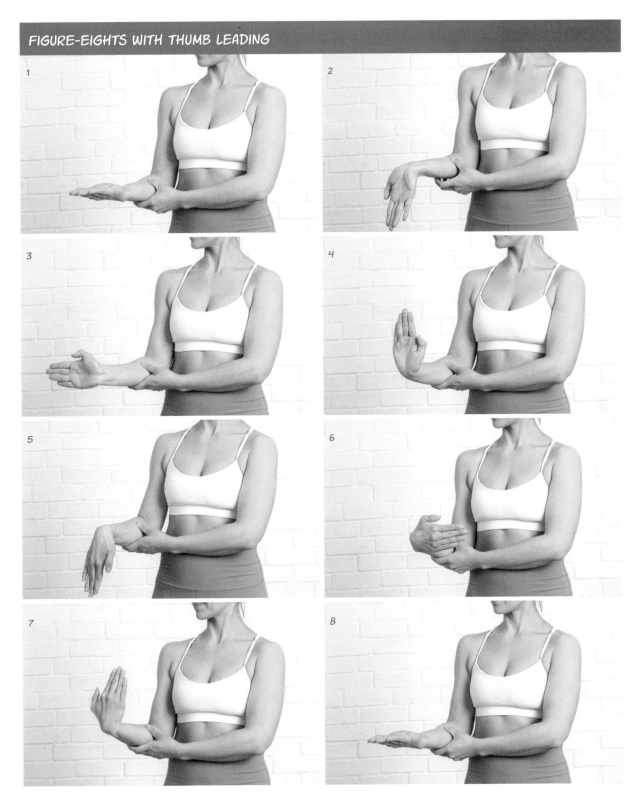

- **Hand figure-eights with thumb leading:** Start with your palm facing down and your wrist flexed. Turn your hand at the wrist in the direction of the thumb until your fingers point upward. Extend your wrist as if you're high-fiving someone upside down. Turn your hand at the wrist toward your thumb to complete the figure-eight.

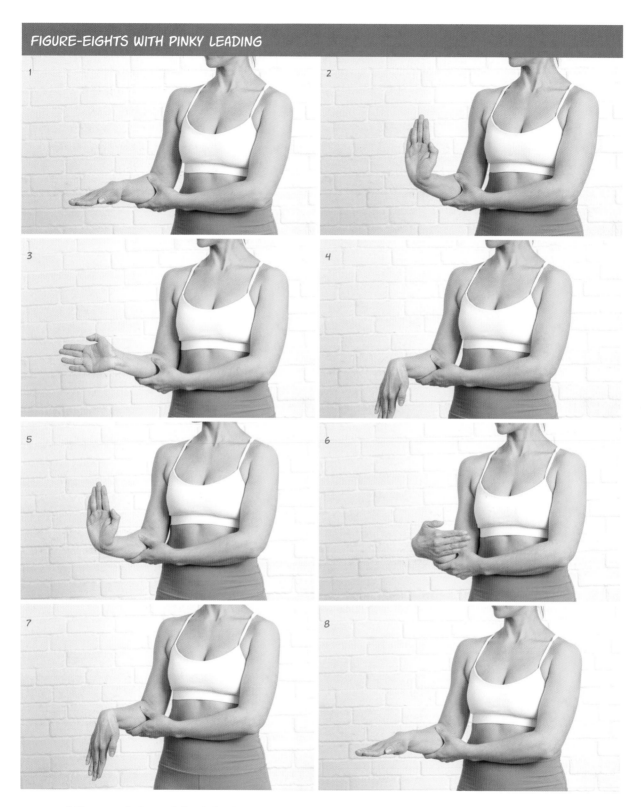

- **Hand figure-eights with pinky leading:** Start with your palm facing up and your wrist flexed. Turn your hand at the wrist in the direction of your little finger until your fingers are pointing down. Extend your wrist as if you're high-fiving someone. Turn your hand at the wrist toward your little finger to complete the figure-eight.

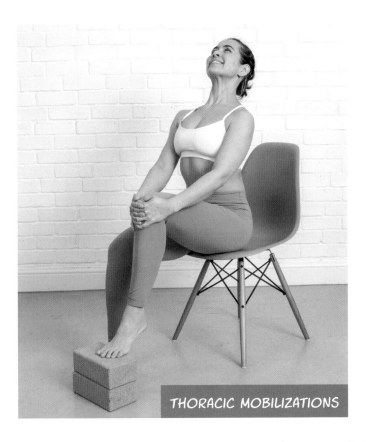

THORACIC MOBILIZATIONS

- **Thoracic spine mobilizations:** Sit in a chair and place one leg on a low stool or a pair of blocks. Interlace your fingers around the front of your knee and round your upper back. Then reverse the movement by extending your upper back. Keep your neck in neutral and don't let your shoulders do all the movement.

If you were to go on a romantic date with your cerebellum, you'd better be on form. For the cerebellum to stay engaged, it needs novelty, unpredictability, and challenge.[131] Therefore, varying the movements you try as you seek to make them harder and more complex will get your cerebellum to fall in love with you. There are many ways to do this. For example:

- Instead of just doing straight up-and-down lunges, add hip circles.

- Instead of doing plain push-ups, add neck circles.

- Instead of doing a static yoga pose, add wrist figure-eights.

These are only three examples, but there are literally millions of exercises that you can modify to light up your cerebellum.

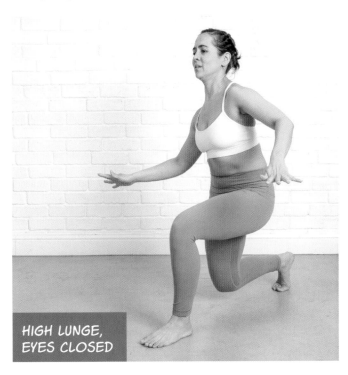

HIGH LUNGE, EYES CLOSED

The cerebellum is also a stickler for detail, so be sure to involve some level of accuracy in your training.[131] We mentioned juggling earlier, but you can also give yourself specific targets, like landing a jump on a specific spot or tapping the tip of your nose with your index finger during a high lunge.

One last suggestion is to give yourself some balance challenges.[132,149] For example, stand on one leg and try moving your gaze, keep your gaze steady and try moving your head around, or try moving on the six coordinates of a compass (up, down, side-to-side, and on the diagonal).

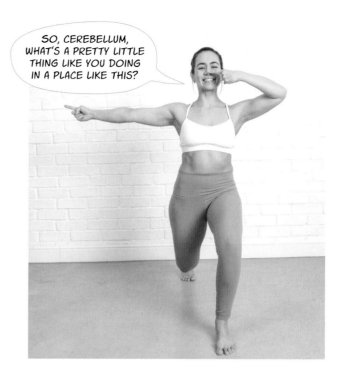

POSTURAL SWAY

Something we often see when we watch members of our Bendy Family move is something called *postural sway*, marked by an uncontrolled sway in the movement pathway. Although weakness could be the villain in question, it's more accurate to work on the higher-order balance systems, such as the vestibular system and cerebellum, which sets the tone of the extensors, that sweet booty-licious glute gang, and the rest of the posterior chain.[133]

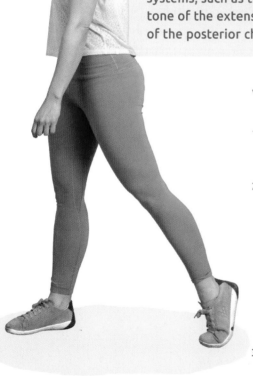

Vestibular Drill

1. Stand with your feet together, close your eyes, and observe how much you sway.

2. Keeping your eyes closed and your feet together, move your head quickly into various positions and hold each one for 10 to 20 seconds.

    – Turn your head left to right
    – Tilt your head left to right
    – Move your head up and down
    – Move your head on the diagonal

3. Repeat the same head positions with a hold while standing on one leg and keeping your eyes open.

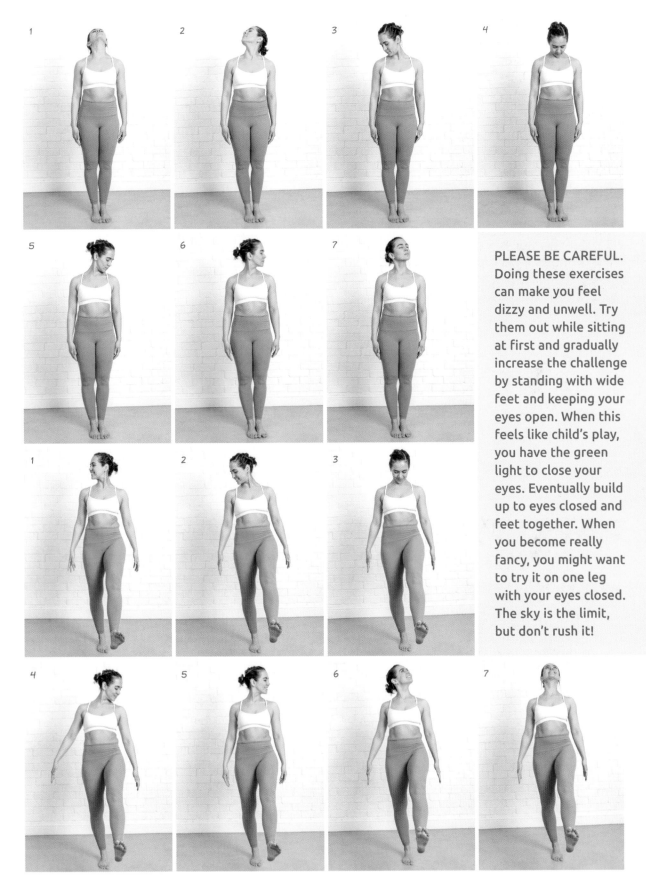

PLEASE BE CAREFUL. Doing these exercises can make you feel dizzy and unwell. Try them out while sitting at first and gradually increase the challenge by standing with wide feet and keeping your eyes open. When this feels like child's play, you have the green light to close your eyes. Eventually build up to eyes closed and feet together. When you become really fancy, you might want to try it on one leg with your eyes closed. The sky is the limit, but don't rush it!

Perturbation

We keep banging on about this nifty trick because it's especially great for the hypermobile fam—even more so if you're like the two of us and your body is always leaning to one side or the other.

Grab a stretchy band and step inside it; then connect it to an external object so that it's pulling you off-center (perturbation) while you bust out your shapes—for example, lunges.[134] Celest's body is always leaning to the right, so she attaches the band to something on her right side, thereby forcing her body to pull to the left. This helps activate all the weak muscles in her body that often struggle to turn on. If you're like her, make sure to use this trick and attach the band to the side to which your body leans. If you don't share this strange phenomenon, you can still use the band strategy but alternate sides.

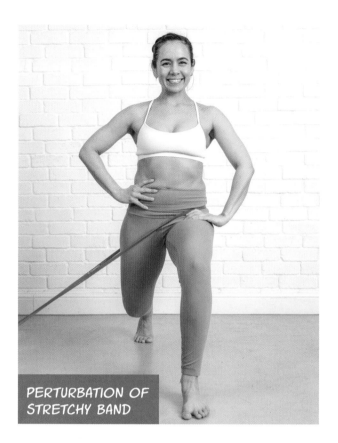

PERTURBATION OF STRETCHY BAND

DEVELOPING MUSCULAR STRENGTH IN YOUR POSTERIOR CHAIN

To get your posterior chain alive and well again, you need to hit it from every angle. The first step is to be mindful of your glutes while you're spending time on your belly in a position commonly referred to as "tummy time." This is a colloquial term used to describe placing a baby in a prone position (on their tummy) to help develop their postural muscles. We tend to use this body position while playing on our phones, reading a book, or sunbathing.

When you're in this position, you might feel your ribs flaring and your lower back tightening, so try squeezing your butt, especially when there is additional spinal extension.[136] Here, you especially rely on Gluteus Maximus to step into his gladiatorial glory, shifting the focus away from your back muscles.[125]

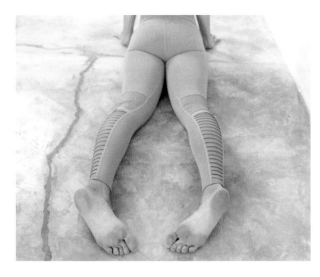
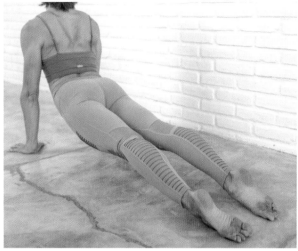

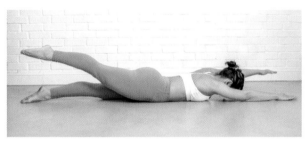
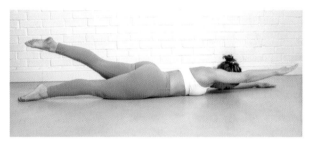

If you want to incorporate this concept into your training, lie on your belly and practice unsupported cobra with Team Gluteus *on* like Donkey Kong.

You can also add a Pilates exercise called Swimmers. You kick your legs up, one at a time, to get your hips into extension from Team Gluteus. Although this move is necessary when swimming, it's even more applicable in walking.

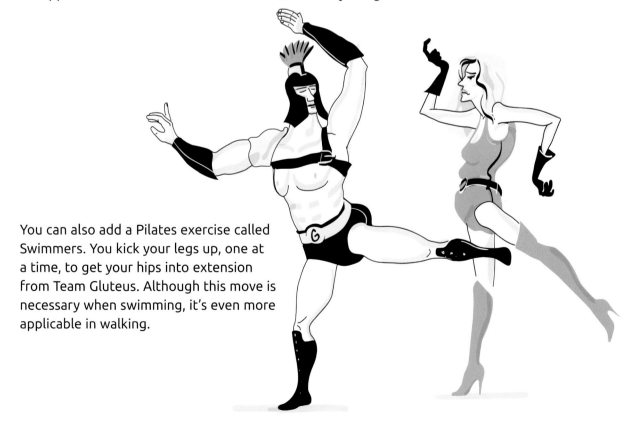

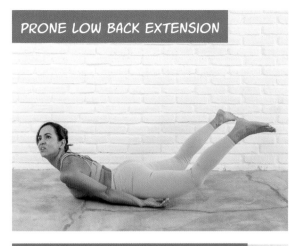

PRONE LOW BACK EXTENSION

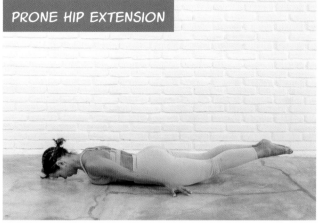

PRONE HIP EXTENSION

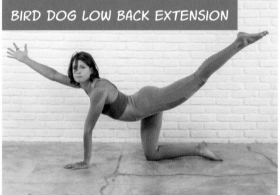

BIRD DOG LOW BACK EXTENSION

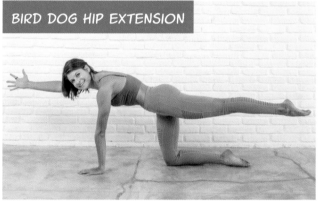

BIRD DOG HIP EXTENSION

It's worth focusing your extension efforts on your butt (for hip extension) and upper back (for thoracic extension) instead of letting your lower back do all the bending. It's not that your lower back shouldn't bend at all; you just don't want to rely on it in isolation.

The next step is to keep your posterior chain engaged while performing lifting tasks or resistance training.[124] If the gym is scary, uncharted territory for you and you're not ready for it, then start at home using resistance bands to do deadlifts, single-leg deadlifts, and overhead squats. You can even just stand tall with a resistance band looped over your shoulder and under your foot to load your postural muscles (see page 92).[135] If you want to add in weights at home, start with a water bottle and progressively build up to water cooler!

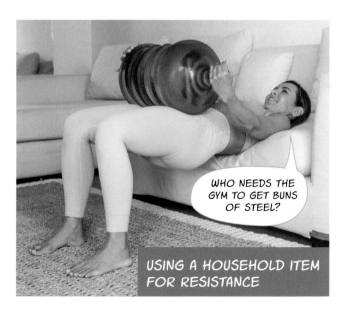

WHO NEEDS THE GYM TO GET BUNS OF STEEL?

USING A HOUSEHOLD ITEM FOR RESISTANCE

Once you feel that your posterior chain and stability muscles are part of the crime-busting team, it's time to banish the villains by venturing to the gym, if possible.[124] Remember, it's important to mimic what you would be doing in nature (the ultimate villain killer), so adding a few pulling and lifting actions to your workouts will give your body a little taste of what it has evolved to do.

The following are some of our favorite villain-killer exercises.

Squats

In the wild, our ancestors would squat for almost everything, from their morning dump to the afternoon hunt. To destroy Sedentary Seductress's evil plans, we need to squat and squat well.[137] Here are some tips to start your squatting journey:

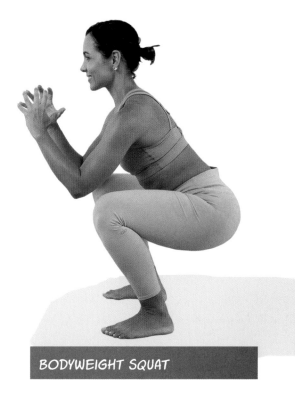

BODYWEIGHT SQUAT

- Position your feet a little wider than hip width apart.

- Turn your toes slightly outward.

- Keep your body upright.

- Keep your eyes forward.

- Turn on your deep neck flexors.

- Consciously squeeze your butt throughout the entire movement.

- Add torque (see page 122).

Our description is not the only way to squat. What we've shared is just a start to elevate your mind-body link. In nature, your body would move around in the squat position in an infinite number of ways. Therefore, brave Bendy, once you've mastered the rules, feel free to break them and go all Picasso on us. The only thing we ask is that you break the rules *with your muscles supporting your joints.* It's very easy to turn them off and overstress your ligaments.[138]

You can also try these squat variations:

- Feet turned out

- Feet turned in

- One foot turned out and the other turned in

- One foot in front of the other combining the foot options above

Resistance Band Squat Variations

We highly recommend adding resistance to your squatting routine. Here are a few suggestions for how to use a band to up your squatting game.

Spinal Lengthening

We previously hinted at this exercise being a goodie for TVA, but the truth is, it's good for all of your postural muscles.[136,139]

- Step one foot inside the band and loop it over your opposite shoulder, a bit like you've won a beauty contest and you're wearing a sash.

- Keeping your spine long and your feet hip width apart, practice doing small knee bends.

- Add rotation. Bend your knees as you rotate, straighten your knees, and then turn back to the front. Switch the band to the other side and repeat in the other direction.

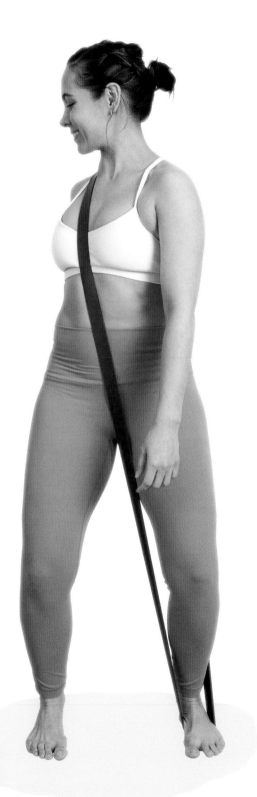

SPINAL LENGTHENING

Lateral Pull Squats

Loop the band around something sturdy and either step inside it or hold the free end in your hands as you do your squats, adding perturbation. This technique is also a great way to spice up lunges and deadlifts.

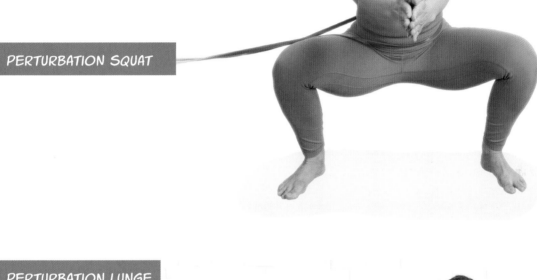

PERTURBATION SQUAT

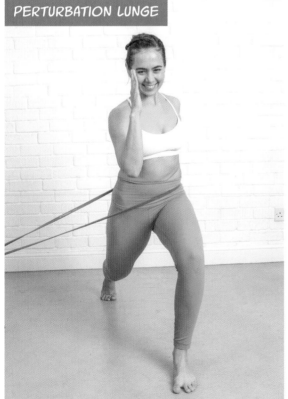

PERTURBATION LUNGE

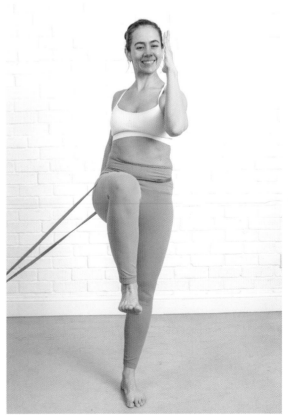

Deadlifts

Deadlifts are another prime example of what would happen in nature. To survive, our forebears would lift heavy loads such as food, water, shelter-building materials, and children.[141] To mimic these actions, deadlifts are awesome exercises to bring into your routine. Here are some tips to deadlift well:

- Start with a tall spine.

- Turn on your glutes and keep them engaged as you bend to reach for the weight or resistance band.

- Make sure to initiate the movement by shifting your hips back. This means your butt will stick out all sassy, and your spine will be in neutral, which places the load on your glutes. It's not the end of the world if your back rounds, but you want your glutes to be the main driver of the exercise.

- Engage your glutes throughout the entire movement, even on the way down.

- Keep your shoulders pulled back to mimic a "pull" action.

- Maintain activation in your deep neck flexors.

- Add torque (see page 122).

No need to always follow these rules. They are just the starting point; they're by no means the finish line.

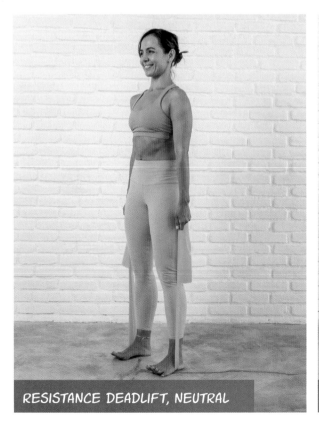

RESISTANCE DEADLIFT, NEUTRAL

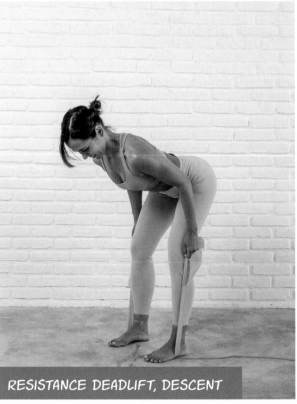

RESISTANCE DEADLIFT, DESCENT

Single-Leg Deadlifts

The single-leg deadlift is not a movement necessarily found in nature, but we love it because it enables Emperor Gluteus Maximus Aurelius and Sassy Stability Agent Gluteus Medius to slay Trendelenburg (see page 112).[142] Follow these steps:

1. Stand on one leg, keeping your opposite knee as high to your chest as possible without compensation. (Compensation might be leaning back or bending your supporting leg.) Keep both hips level to get your gluteus medius firing.

2. Hinge from your hip by sticking your butt out (anterior pelvic tilt), maintain a tall spine, and extend the lifted leg back, parallel to the floor.

3. Engage your glute max (the round part of your butt) throughout the movement.

4. Add torque (see page 122).

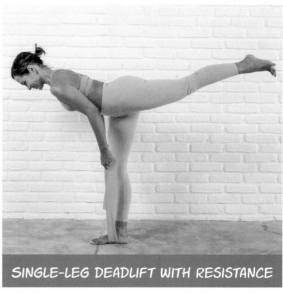

SINGLE-LEG DEADLIFT WITH RESISTANCE

Again, once you're strong and can move smoothly in and out of these movement pathways under load, we highly encourage you to get creative with your movement and break all the rules. Apart from the holy grail—don't hang in your ligaments—you can color outside the lines.

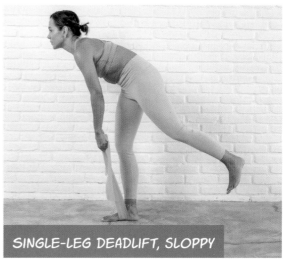

SINGLE-LEG DEADLIFT, SLOPPY

If you've been working a desk job and binge-watching Netflix, these exercises might make your muscles ache. Sitting leaves your glute max turned off and in a lengthened position for most of the day. Emperor Gluteus Maximus Aurelius is literally hanging on by a thread.[140] Gone are its gladiatorial glory days with the coliseum crowd cheering for its rotund juiciness. Getting your glutes working again will take patience and time, but it'll also ensure that your lax joints will be well supported! So please, don't skip leg day.

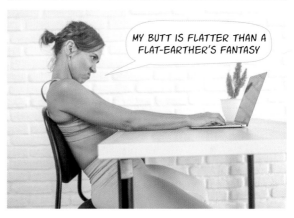

MY BUTT IS FLATTER THAN A FLAT-EARTHER'S FANTASY

WALKING

Walking, also known as the gait cycle, is a complex bodily process of using momentum and activation to create motion. We want to zoom in on the role of your glute max (but without going into insomnia-curing detail). Remember, G-Max enables hip extension, which is an important action for walking because we use this action to propel ourselves forward.[124] However, some people's glutes are so weak that extension isn't happening from the hip; instead, it's transferred to the spine. Although this adaptation serves the purpose of getting you from point A to point B, it's not ideal.[143] See, the hip is a *huge* joint, and the glutes are the biggest muscles in the body. Our bodies require a good 10,000 to 15,000 steps per day to operate functionally, so relying on these larger body parts makes sense.

If this workaround continues for a short while, there shouldn't be much consequence. Alternative strategies exist to save the day if and when needed. The trouble is that the lumbar spine requires stability, so if the adaptation continues for months or years, the excessive, unnatural use might put strain on the connections of the spine.[143] Not everyone will find this adaptation problematic, but if you do, we have a simple solution: get Team Gluteus to join the party and redirect the load away from your lower back when walking.

Back pain isn't always related to a structural issue in the body. Sometimes emotional stress—and even job satisfaction—can play a role. Always take care of your body, but if what you're doing isn't helping your pain, dig a little deeper.

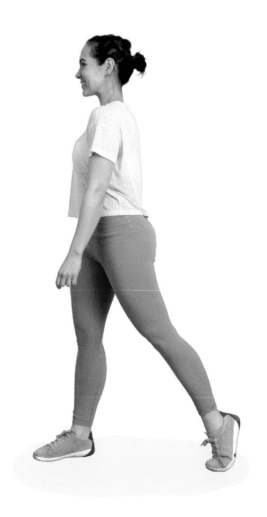

YOUR FEET AND GLUTE MAX

Still on the topic of gait, let's look at how your feet—and more specifically your shoes—can contribute to and exacerbate glute max weakness.

Shoes have the nifty job of keeping your feet safe. Some footwear takes that responsibility very seriously, so much so that it restricts all movement in the feet and especially in the toes because of a rigid sole that stays flat with each step (or, more specifically, with each push-off). Walking with the glute max pushing the hips into extension means that your toes need a lot of mobility to allow your legs to reach behind you. If your feet can't move naturally—if they're caged into a single shape—your knees bend prematurely and your legs don't get pushed back far enough for the glute max to kick in during the push-off phase in your gait cycle.[144] Compare the images below and notice how the push-off phase is limited when the foot is kept in a rigid shape.[145] If you don't have the ability to extend your toes, Gluteus Maximus Aurelius will think that you don't need his services anymore, so he'll go back to watching *Friends* on repeat.[146] Now, if you wear a cute pair of stiff shoes once in a while, that's OK! But remember, your little feet have been squeezed into rigid shoes since you were much younger, which means that it's going to take some doing to rewire your walking pattern and get Gluteus Maximus Aurelius to do his job.

> We think minimal shoes are a great investment. However, they should come with a warning label. Suddenly transitioning from a cushioned, rigid sole to barefoot shoes is asking for trouble. You need time to adapt to the differences. We recommend making the transition progressively (there's that word again) over a three- to six-month period. In addition, strengthen your foot's myofascial system so your foot learns to support itself without relying on the shoe; see the exercises in Chapter 8.[122]

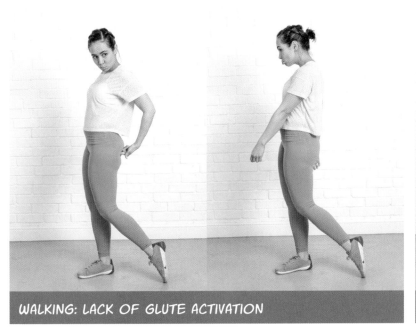

WALKING: LACK OF GLUTE ACTIVATION

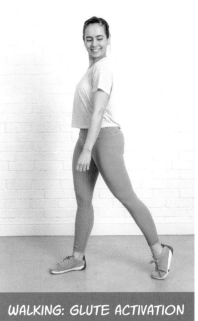

WALKING: GLUTE ACTIVATION

HAMSTRINGS

The hamstrings are a sidekick to Team Gluteus that often tags along and helps Team Glutes save the day. But if you're a part of the human family, chances are furniture is supporting your butt for a large portion of the day, which is having an adverse effect on your hamstrings. (Sedentary Seductress is doing an evil laugh this very second as she watches the citizens of the world get cozy in their seats.) Tight hamstrings are often a reason people decide to start yoga: "My hamstrings feel tight. *I KNOW,* I'll take up yoga!" Bendies like us, on the other hand, muse, "I'm a black belt in toe touching; I should take up yoga."

Often, that first experience with yoga is the moment hypermobile people discover that, contrary to their long-held belief, they're not totally useless at all movement disciplines. In fact, in their very first class, the teacher might praise them for having a "beautiful practice."

"Me? Beautiful?" the novice muses. "How are my movements 'beautiful'? I remember coming in last for everything in school." But that look of certainty from the teacher, the knowing nods and raised eyebrows, all feed the deep-seated need to be loved and accepted and part of a gang of equally "beautiful" people who can also touch foot to head without any real effort.

This praise is, of course, not a problem as long as adequate biomechanical knowledge is passed on to the Bendy Person—knowledge that will equip them to keep their body safe from excessively straining passively into their joints. Sadly, this education isn't the norm right now. Yoga loves the same repetitive movements, and the movement pattern that yogis execute more than any other is the forward fold.

Excessive forward folds often lead to a syndrome affectionately named "yoga butt." This issue develops when a practitioner has done so many forward folds, with little strength training, that the upper attachments of the muscles (the tendons) succumb to injury.[40]

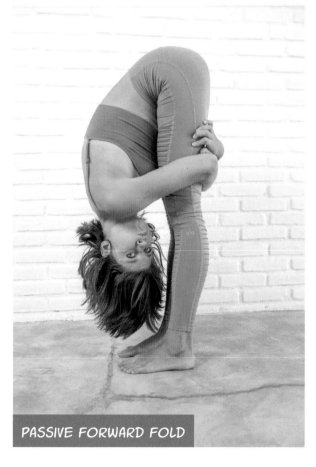

PASSIVE FORWARD FOLD

Forward folds are actually quite safe when they're cued correctly. Flexi family, pay close attention: you need to protect your ligaments and tendons by using the myofascial system through *activation*. In a forward fold, this means engaging your butt and hamstrings. At the bottom of the movement, avoid pulling yourself into a deeper range; instead, use your active strength.[147]

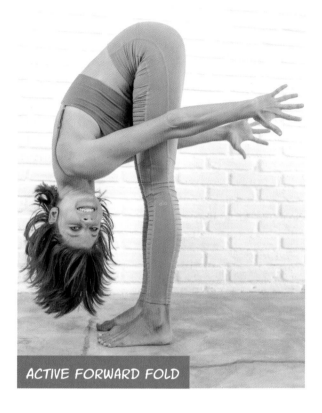

ACTIVE FORWARD FOLD

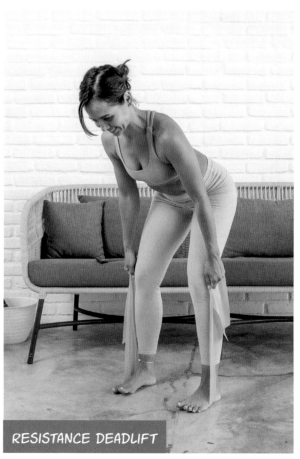

RESISTANCE DEADLIFT

Ultimately, your hamstrings have evolved to lift loads. We neglected lifting for years, so our hamstrings were long and thin (and sore) from too much time spent stretching. Finally, we saw the light and incorporated deadlifts—which are arguably the most important exercise any hypermobile person can ever incorporate! Deadlifts mimic lifting and therefore activate the posterior chain through load, which can help reverse the adverse effects from doing too many forward folds. They strengthen the tendons (attachments) of the hamstrings and therefore help prevent and rehab yoga butt. When you perform deadlifts with a lengthened spine, you progressively overload your glutes and hamstrings so that they can support your body for many more hours in a day.[141]

CHAPTER 7:

PROXIMAL STABILITY

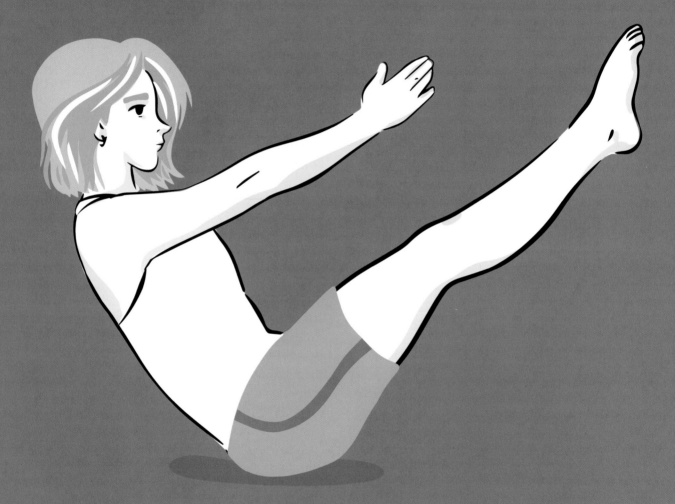

If you had to consciously control all of your body all of the time, it would be mentally exhausting—and probably unsustainable. The good news is that this isn't necessary when your proximal stabilizers (the larger stability muscles closer to your spine) are working reflexively. In this chapter, we explore the stability muscles that we feel all Bendies should know about and pay some attention to: Serratus Shadow Wing Anterior and Sassy Stability Agent Gluteus Medius.

SHOULDERS

You know how you can put sunscreen on even the most (seemingly) unreachable parts of your body? This special superpower is courtesy of the extraordinary range of motion available at your shoulder joint. However, it is important to remember that "with great sunscreen application power comes great responsibility."

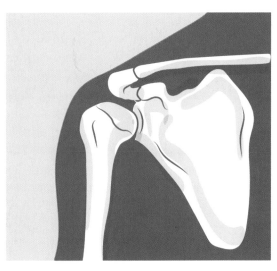

You see, as with all the other joints we've covered, we need to be mindful not to overdo end-range stretches so that we don't compromise our ligaments. In the shoulder, this effect is magnified because the shoulder socket is disproportionately small, which provides less structural support for the large head of the arm bone (humerus).

The result is favorable because you have less bony occlusion getting in the way of your sunscreen application, but the downside is that shoulders tend to be unstable joints that rely heavily on strong, balanced muscles to support such a large range of motion.[154]

SERRATUS SHADOW WING ANTERIOR

One of the most important, yet neglected, shoulder-saving superheroes is Serratus Shadow Wing Anterior.[155] The shoulder is the most mobile and complex joint in the body, whether a person has the superpower of hypermobility or not. But hypermobility does mean we have to put extra time and attention into our muscular strength and pay special attention to honing the skills of Serratus Shadow Wing Anterior. This soft-spoken, but not-to-be-underestimated, muscle superhero is like a hidden wing in the shadow of your arm. It comes from the ribs at the front of the body, wrapping around the side of your ribs and under your armpit to attach on the underside of your shoulder blade (scapula). She's a superhero muscle, for sure, because she enables the scapula to lie flush on the ribs. When she's doing her thing and the scapula is being pulled into a good position, the stability and mobility of the joint as a whole are improved.[155]

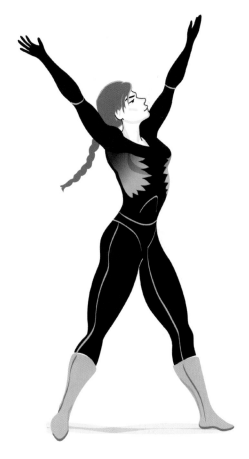

The challenge is that the serratus anterior can be stubborn and difficult to activate, so you have to get to it from every angle. Not only must you strengthen it with targeted exercises, but you also have to retrain your nervous system to keep the serratus anterior stabilized when you are carrying a heavy suitcase, doing the conga, or fetching a teacup from the cupboard.[156] Basically, anytime you're doing anything, this muscle should be working reflexively to keep your shoulder blade in a biomechanically sound position.[155]

How can you tell if your serratus anterior isn't working? Well, the first thing to do is to somehow get a view of your back. You can try a double mirror or use a tripod to film yourself. Get naked and take a look at your shoulder blades. If they're coming away from your rib cage, this is a clear indication that your serratus anterior needs some attention. It's also worth filming yourself or finding a friend with a little anatomy knowledge to have a look at your shoulder blades while you're doing your favorite movement discipline. Use these tools to get feedback about what your scapulae are doing while you're moving. If they tend to stick up off of your rib cage, your serratus anterior needs some targeted exercises to get it stronger.[157]

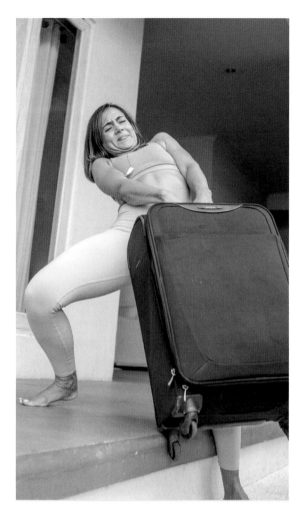

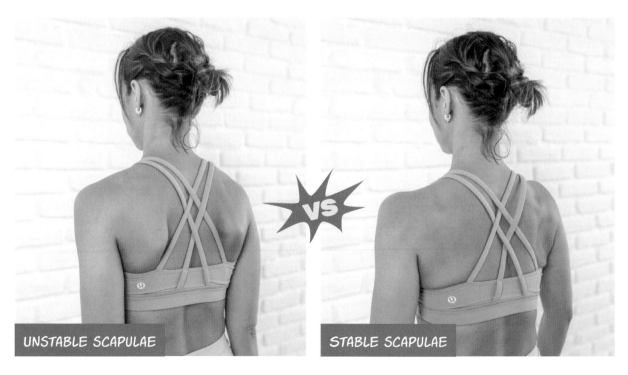

UNSTABLE SCAPULAE

STABLE SCAPULAE

At first, we need to teach our serratus to control a movement known as *scapulohumeral rhythm*.[158] This fancy term simply means that wherever your arm goes, so should your shoulder blade. For example, when you're reaching up to retrieve a teacup from a high shelf, your shoulder blade should glide up. As you're bringing the teacup down, the scapula should come down, too. The serratus is controlling the pathway of the scapulae. In the next sections, we suggest some exercises you can use to help strengthen the serratus.

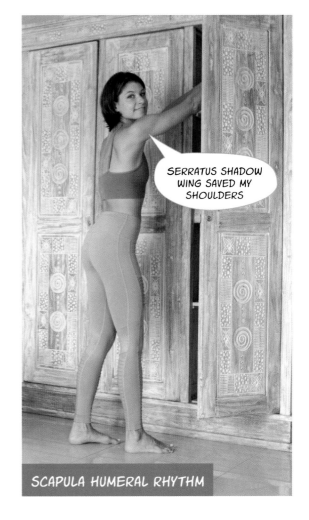

SERRATUS SHADOW WING SAVED MY SHOULDERS

SCAPULA HUMERAL RHYTHM

Have you ever been to a yoga or Pilates class where the teacher cued you to draw your shoulder blades down as you lifted your arms up? This is an old-skool cue that came from the dance world for aesthetic reasons. It is not based on sound biomechanical reasoning, and this cue does not have your shoulders' best interests at heart. Please move your scapulae![157] Keeping them fixed in place is bad news!

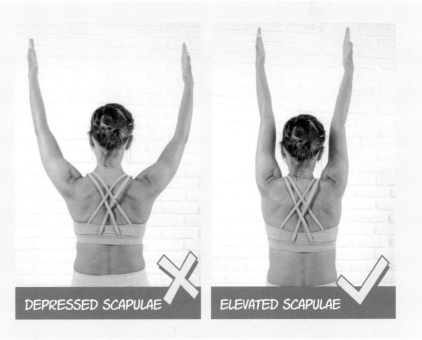

DEPRESSED SCAPULAE

ELEVATED SCAPULAE

Wall Glides

To teach your serratus to control the scapulae for reaching motions, face a wall and place your forearms on the wall. Maintain a long spine as you glide your forearms up the wall into a *V* shape. Notice whether you allow your ribs to flare open or your neck to collapse. Work on keeping a tall spine from the crown of your head and maintain a stable body.[157] It's worth filming your back and then reviewing the video to see if your scapulae stay on the straight and narrow as your arms glide up and down. Ideally, you want to see the scapulae moving without losing control and popping off of your back.

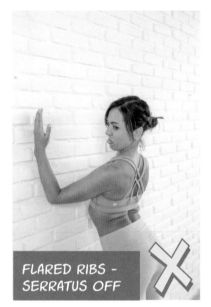

FLARED RIBS -
SERRATUS OFF ✗

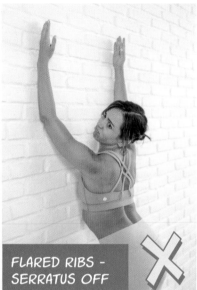

FLARED RIBS -
SERRATUS OFF ✗

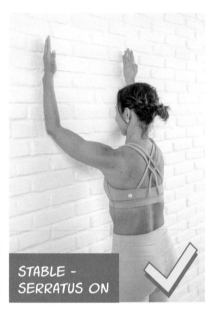

STABLE -
SERRATUS ON ✓

Serratus anterior is a huge muscle that is comprised of upper, mid, and lower fibers.159 Next, we describe how to get all three sections of your wings stronger.

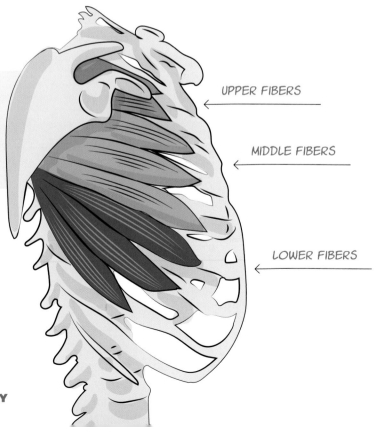

UPPER FIBERS

MIDDLE FIBERS

LOWER FIBERS

Upper Fibers of Serratus

Place two blocks under your hands and perform elevation and depression of the scapulae. Push down, allowing the scapulae to glide down your back. Reverse the movement to let your shoulders move slowly with control toward your ears. Keep the scapulae flat on your back throughout the movement.

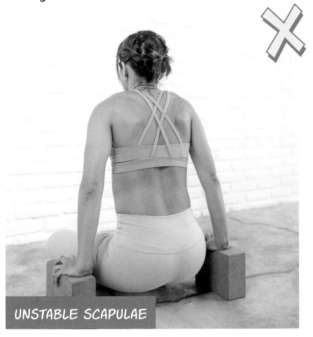

UNSTABLE SCAPULAE

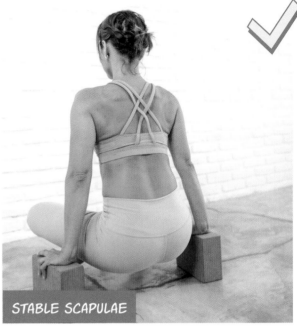

STABLE SCAPULAE

Mid Fibers

Next, target the mid fibers by coming into a plank position and gliding the scapulae toward each other into retraction and then away from each other into protraction. Be careful that the movement isn't translated to other parts of your body, such as your head or belly collapsing. Keep everything strong and solid and isolate the movements to your scapulae gliding.

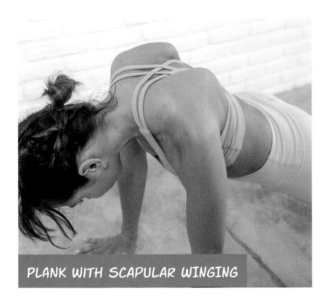

PLANK WITH SCAPULAR WINGING

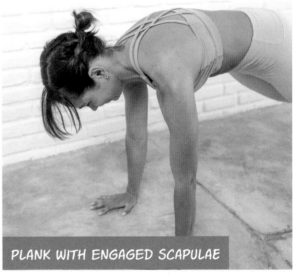

PLANK WITH ENGAGED SCAPULAE

Lower Fibers

Here, we revisit scapular elevation and depression. Place your forearms on the floor and interlace your fingers. Come into a headstand position but keep your toes on the floor, with your hips up. Push down on your forearms to allow your head to lift away from the floor. Keep your front ribs in and round your upper back. Then control the descent until your head gently touches the floor again.

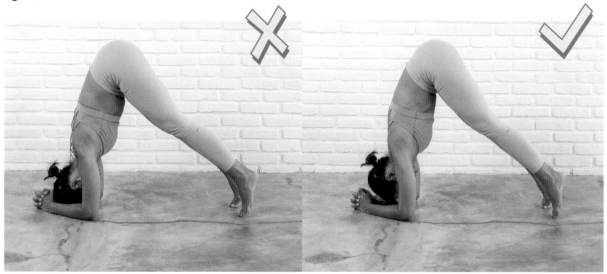

Camshafts

To be honest, even though we want to educate you about the glory of the serratus, it is impossible to isolate a single muscle. The body just doesn't work like that. The truth is that when you're performing these exercises, other muscles are getting involved, too. That's why we especially love camshafts (affectionately named after the mechanics of train wheels; see the image below). This is a genius exercise because it helps activate all the muscles that control the movements of the shoulder blade.

Stand tall, lift your arms parallel to the floor, and open them out at a 45-degree angle. Keep your arms straight as you move your scapulae in circular motions, much like the camshafts on the wheels of a train. Perform these scapular circles both forward and backward.

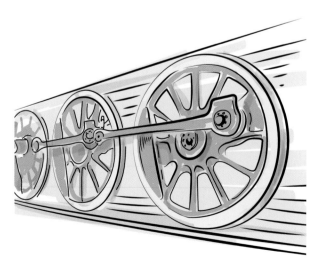

You can add a resistance band to the mix to spice things up. Loop the band around your back and secure it to something to one side of your body. With the other arm holding the band, reach forward and perform the camshaft, one shoulder at a time.

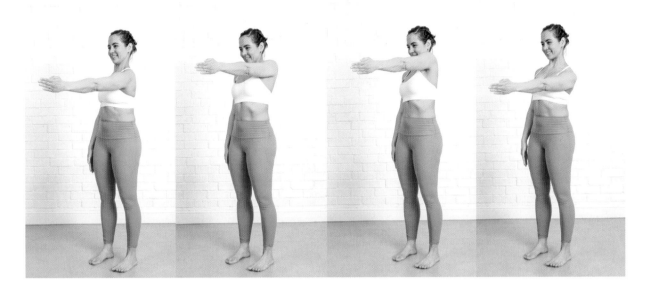

Carrying a Heavy Bag

We're sure the rest of the population would laugh at us if they knew the intention behind this next drill, but bear with us. When hypermobile people carry anything of substantial weight, it is not uncommon for them to allow the weight of the object to distract the shoulder joint and overstretch the ligaments.[38]

To train the stability of the shoulder in this instance, loop a stretchy band under your feet and hold one end in each hand. Practice letting the stretchy band "win" by pulling your shoulder down to the ground. Then resist the weight of the band by turning on your serratus muscle. Please note: This is *not* pulling your shoulder blades up to your ears. Your shoulder blades should stay at the same height, but the lowest point should make a scooping motion under your armpit.

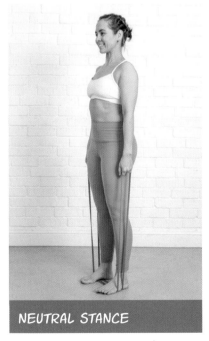

NEUTRAL STANCE

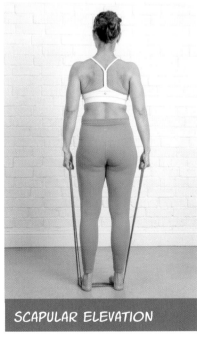

SCAPULAR ELEVATION

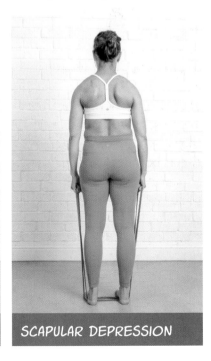

SCAPULAR DEPRESSION

Shoulder Circles

We've gone into a lot of detail about getting the scapulae to be stable, but now we would like to shift our focus a little lower to the ball-and-socket joint. Remember that this is the joint that's prone to instability, so it's worth getting the neural mapping in tip-top shape.[155,159]

While you're standing, move one arm so it's parallel to the floor and point it out at a 45-degree angle. Now circle the arm from the head of the humerus, as shown in the images below. Imagine touching the inside edge of a small hoop that's encircling your upper arm.

To add resistance, loop a band around your back and extend the other arm forward while holding the band. Then draw your circles.

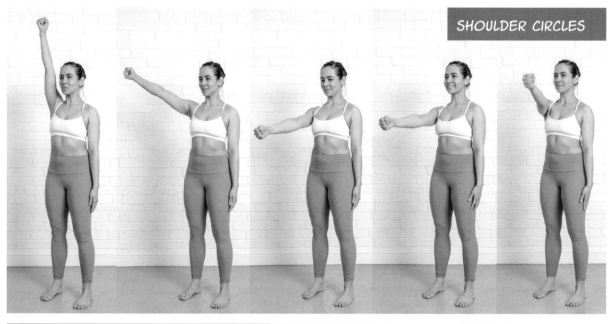

SHOULDER CIRCLES

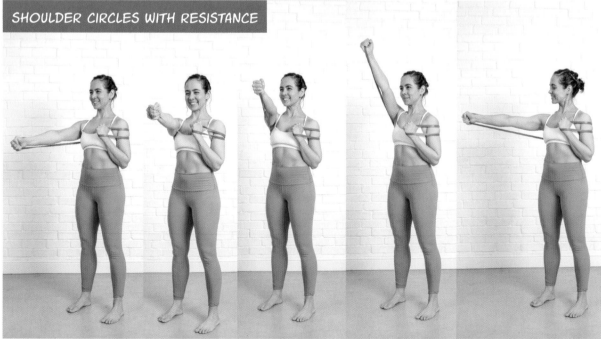

SHOULDER CIRCLES WITH RESISTANCE

Shoulder Figure-Eights

This exercise is similar to the previous one. You move from the ball and socket of the shoulder joint to draw a figure-eight with your arm. It may help to imagine you have a pen in your hand.

Up the ante and add a resistance band as you did for the shoulder circles. Loop the band around your back and secure it with one hand. Then draw your figure-eights and feel the magic!

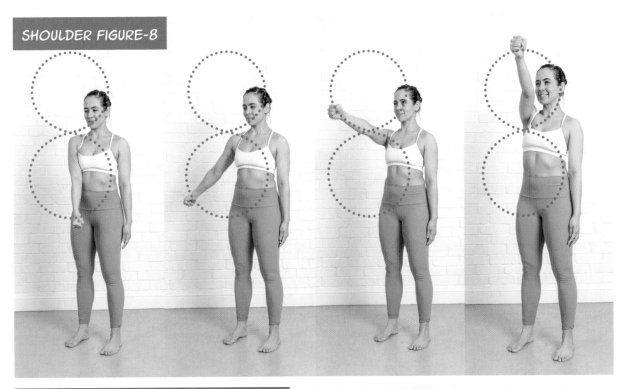

SHOULDER FIGURE-8

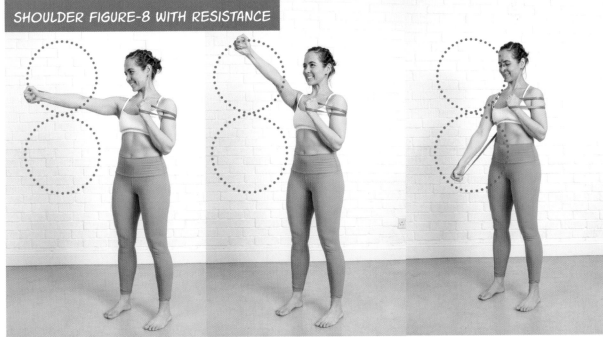

SHOULDER FIGURE-8 WITH RESISTANCE

REFLEXIVE SHOULDER STABILITY

Although targeted exercises are great, the real shoulder-saving super stuff comes through *reflexive activation,* which is useful because it happens without thought. This is where we love movements that stimulate the brain stem.[27]

Remember earlier in the book when we talked about Big Daddy Brain and explained how doing a movement with one side (like grabbing a cup of coffee) requires reflexive stability to flood the opposite side of the body? (See page 45.) Those stability commands come from the brain stem in an attempt to keep you from falling over.[27,161] You can take advantage of this brain hack in your training.

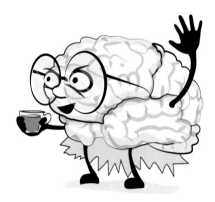

Position yourself on all fours on the floor and stabilize one side as the other arm performs a unique movement pattern, such as a shoulder circle or horizontal row. You can add weights or a resistance band so the moving side has more load, which increases the amount of reflexive stability needed on the opposite side.[160,161]

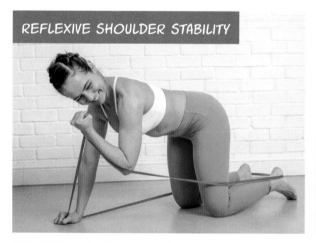

REFLEXIVE SHOULDER STABILITY

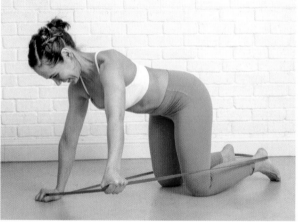

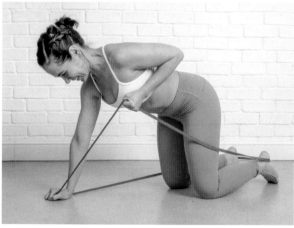

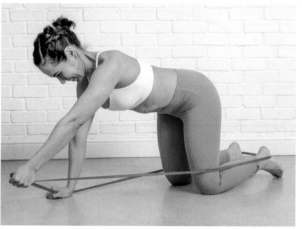

PELVIC STABILITY

We feel so incredibly passionate about Sassy Stability Agent Gluteus Medius (aka Agent M) that we are considering building shrines to her in our homes, complete with creepy photos of strangers whose glute meds are well developed. This muscle does a plethora of awesome stability work on your pelvis and legs. But, as you've probably guessed, the glute med becomes deconditioned due to the lack of variety in our movement patterns. Sorry if we sound like a broken record here. The result is strange compensatory adaptations that often load the joints in unsustainable ways.[162] Let's take a look at some of the movement patterns that the body defaults to when the glute med is nursing a hangover.

Walking and Single-Leg Balances

One of Sassy Stability Agent Gluteus Medius's main powers is her ability to stabilize the pelvis.[162] Think of the pelvis as a single unit in the shape of a Hula-Hoop. Agent M is in charge of keeping the hoop level, especially when it's time to walk, stand on one leg, bear weight through one side more than the other, or even carry a heavy bag.[163]

Here's a strange but relatable example of Agent M working: When Elastidog decides it's time to mark his well-earned territory, he lines himself up to a vertical object, such as a tree or lamppost.

Then, with all his doggy grace, he lifts his leg and allows his territory-marking juices to flow. His ability to stand on a single back leg and lift the other back leg while maintaining a specific pelvic position (so he doesn't pee on himself) comes from the gluteus medius. If that muscle was weak, his pelvis would collapse toward his standing leg, which would then be wet with urine.

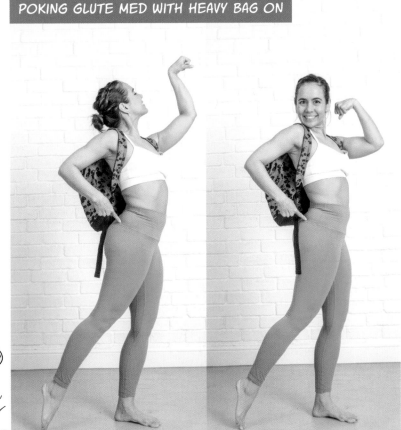

POKING GLUTE MED WITH HEAVY BAG ON

As you lift one leg in preparation to walk, your glute med fires and stabilizes your pelvis. Before you know it, as you take the next step, the other side kicks in to do the same thing. But in most people, Agent M is not as *compos mentis* ("of sound mind") as she should be, and the pelvis dips. This excessive pelvic dipping action is known as Trendelenburg (not a villain name we made up; it really is called that!).[163] You can easily spot this action when you see a model strutting her stuff down a catwalk.

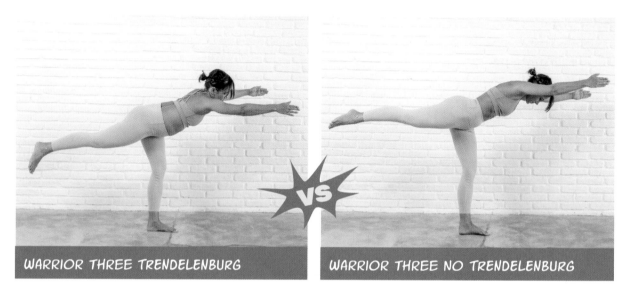

WARRIOR THREE TRENDELENBURG   VS   WARRIOR THREE NO TRENDELENBURG

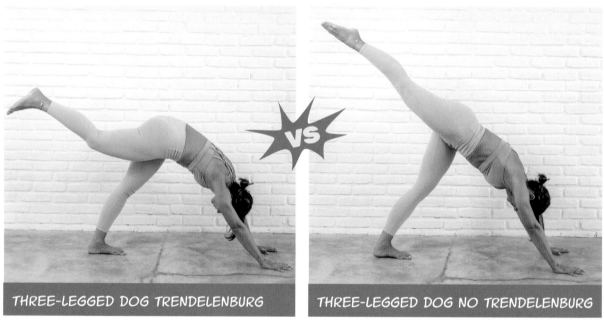

THREE-LEGGED DOG TRENDELENBURG   VS   THREE-LEGGED DOG NO TRENDELENBURG

This collapsing pelvic movement is not ideal, especially for those who are hypermobile, because when it dips, the leg bone (femur) changes its trajectory and often collapses into a strange angle, known as a valgus knee.[163] Our bendy knees often don't have adequate proprioception (sensation signals) to let us know that a valgus knee is bad news.[164] We just carry on until our physiotherapist points out that our strange-looking knees may be contributing to our discomfort.

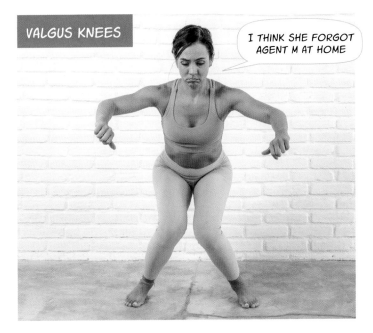

Jump up, take off your pants (if appropriate), go to a mirror, and take a good long look at your lovely legs. Specifically, take a long, hard look at your knees and where they're pointing. If you had laser beams coming out of your knees (the most desirable of all superpowers), where would the lasers point? If your knees rotate inward, there's a strong chance that your glute med needs work.

In addition to giving your pelvis stability, the glute med provides stability for your knees. It does so by keeping your femurs on the straight and narrow rather than letting them go into a valgus collapse. The other benefit is that if the glute med is keeping your long leg bones in check, it's much harder for your bendy joints to move into hyperextension. Hyperextension, like most joint positions, is nothing to fear as long as you don't rely on the ligaments.

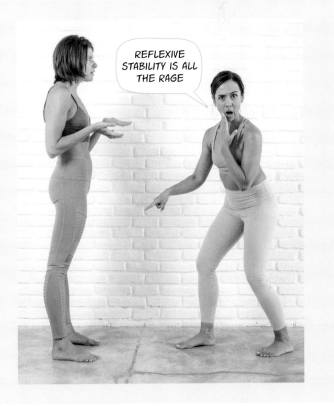

Exercises to Strengthen Agent M

Now that we've looked at the movement patterns that the body defaults to when the glute med needs work, let's look at some exercises to strengthen Agent M.

Clams

Clams are a great starting point for the gluteus medius. Lie on your side and bend your knees. Keep your feet together as you open and close your top leg like a clamshell. To get the most from this exercise, keep your heels connected and your pelvis very still as you move your top leg. Maintain a neutral spine and place your hand on your glute med as you do the exercise so you can feel the activation of the muscle through the pathway.[165]

You might be surprised at how quickly you can feel the burn from such a simple exercise. But you also might be surprised at how quickly you progress and find this exercise too easy. When that happens, get out your booty band to add some more resistance.

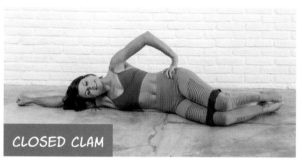
CLOSED CLAM

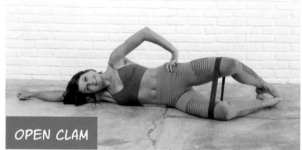
OPEN CLAM

Clams on Crack

Lie on your side just as you did for clams. This time, though, keep your forearm underneath your shoulder. As you clam your legs, push off your forearm and lift your hips. Make sure your spine is in neutral. When you're certain your technique is on point, add a resistance band.

Crab Walk

Place both legs inside a resistance band. Sidestep to the right and left repeatedly. As you do, push your knees out. Also, make sure the leg you're pushing off of has the outer foot and big toe grounded and a strong inner arch.

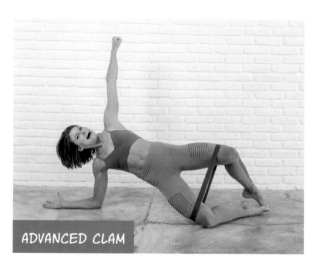
ADVANCED CLAM

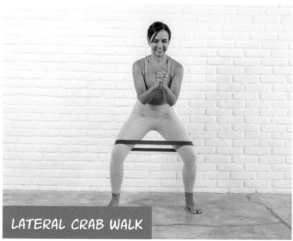
LATERAL CRAB WALK

Zombie Walk

This exercise follows the same principle as the crab walk. Get your legs inside the band and, while driving your knees out against the resistance, take a big diagonal step forward. After taking a few steps, repeat the same number of steps backward, still at a diagonal. Again, make sure the leg you're pushing off of has the outer foot and big toe grounded. Maintain a strong inner arch on that foot, too.

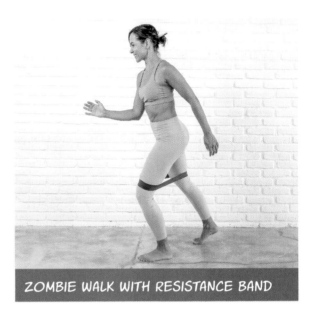

ZOMBIE WALK WITH RESISTANCE BAND

BILATERAL AND UNILATERAL MOVEMENTS

Walking and single-leg balances, as discussed earlier, are known as *unilateral movements*. That means you gotta do one side and then the other. *Bilateral movements*—for example, squats—involve both sides at the same time.

The glute med really comes alive when you're balancing on one leg, but that doesn't mean it's not working when you're on two feet during bilateral movements. Just as your glute med keeps your pelvis level when you're on one side, it also keeps your femur pointing in the right direction when you're on two feet.[162]

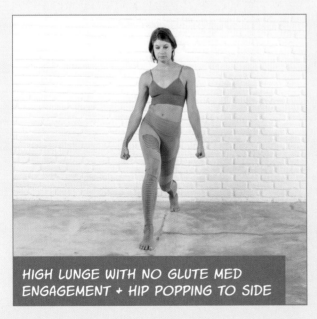

HIGH LUNGE WITH NO GLUTE MED ENGAGEMENT + HIP POPPING TO SIDE

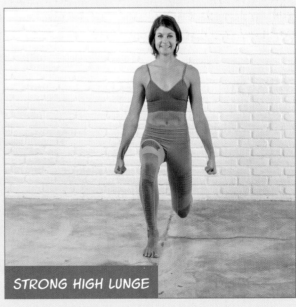

STRONG HIGH LUNGE

Trendelenburg

This one should be named Sassy-burg because it requires a lot of sassy pelvic movement. Stand with one foot on top of a step or block and hover the other leg so your feet are level; in other words, one foot is grounded and the other is floating. The standing leg's gluteus medius is keeping your pelvis level. We want to encourage this gluteus medius to work through full range, so, without bending your knees, allow the pelvis on the standing leg to lower and lift.

Pay attention to the knee of your standing leg and make sure it doesn't collapse into a valgus knee line, with a collapsed inner arch on the foot. The movement should be isolated to the pelvis.

Once you've mastered this movement, allow the standing leg to change its trajectory. Place one foot on the floor and flex the knee of the floating leg to your chest; then perform the Trendelenburg pelvic dips. Or you can extend the leg behind you and then sassy up those hips. If you're feeling really badass, you can even stick an ankle weight on the end of your leg.

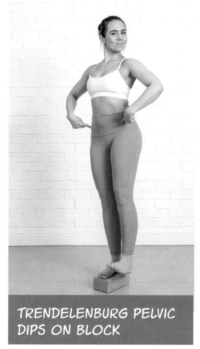

TRENDELENBURG PELVIC DIPS ON BLOCK

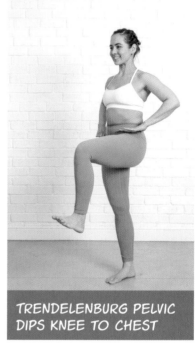

TRENDELENBURG PELVIC DIPS KNEE TO CHEST

Exercises to Strengthen Pelvic Stability

We can move on from the glories of Agent M to look at how we can improve mapping of the pelvis as a whole.

Anterior/Posterior Tilt

Stand with your feet hip width apart and your knees slightly bent. Now tuck your pelvis under (posterior tilt) and then stick your tail bone out (anterior tilt). This is *very* small movement; *don't* move your lower back. Try to isolate the movement into your sacroiliac joints, which is where the pelvis meets the sacrum.[165]

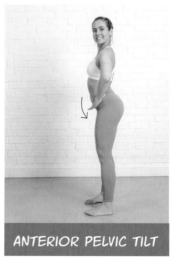

ANTERIOR PELVIC TILT

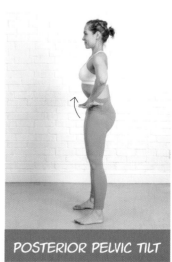

POSTERIOR PELVIC TILT

Side-to-Side Pelvic Tilt

Once you've got the forward-and-back motion down, work on the side-to-side action. This is really tricky for many people, so be patient with yourself.

Stand with your feet together, bend one knee, and allow your pelvis on that same side to drop. The straight leg is supporting the higher side of the pelvis. Now, much like a salsa dancer, shift right and left, letting your pelvis tilt from side to side.

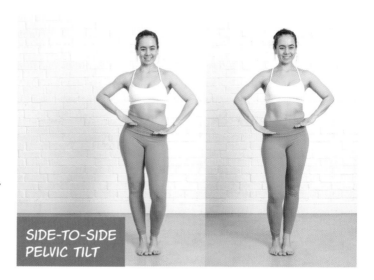

SIDE-TO-SIDE PELVIC TILT

Pelvic Circles

Got the hang of pelvic tilting? Now you can work on getting your pelvis to hit the four corners of a box. Tuck your pelvis (posterior tilt), shift it to one side, stick your butt out (anterior tilt), and then finish the square by shifting your pelvis to the opposite side.

Once you feel confident with this staccato pelvic movement, it's time to connect the four corners of the box in a smooth pelvic circle. You can also step your feet into a variety of patterns as you perform your circles, which challenges your brain on a higher level.[166]

As usual, you can add resistance, too. Step your heel into a stretchy band and pull the band diagonally behind your legs with the end up and over the opposite side of your pelvis. Perform your hip circles with your feet parallel, or play with your foot position. (Don't be shy about experimenting; the more variety, the better.) You also can step your forefoot into the band and bring the band across the fronts of your legs to the opposite hip, as shown on the next page.

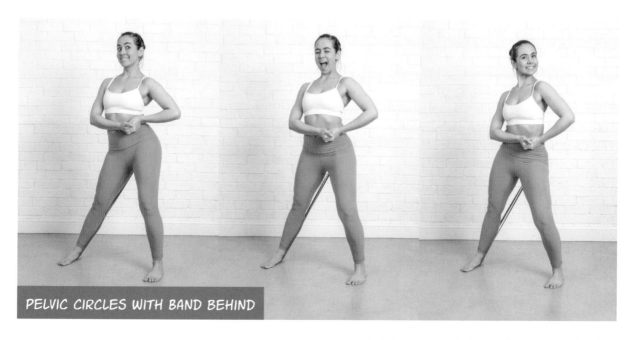

PELVIC CIRCLES WITH BAND BEHIND

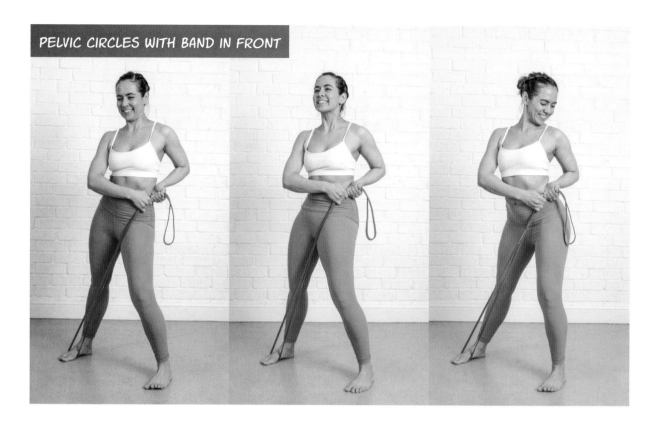

Hip Circles

Next, let's figure out where the maps of your hips are fuzzy. Stand on one leg and lift the opposite leg in front of you as you rotate the lifted leg from the hip (not the foot). First rotate internally and then rotate externally. Which direction felt awkward?

Remember, fuzzy maps could be translated as a threat to the brain, so it's worth getting things sharp and in focus. With that in mind, whichever hip position feels strange is the hip position you should use to perform the next exercise. We call this the *rehab position.*

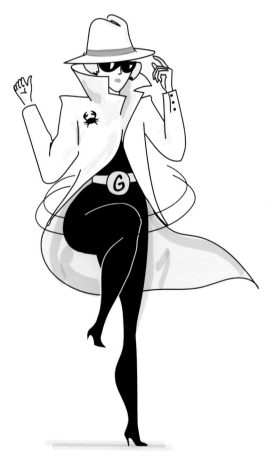

In Celest's body, internal rotation makes her feel like she's sitting alone in a bar without her phone, so she will demo the exercises with internal rotation as her rehab position. But please take a moment to figure out what *your* rehab position is.

Stand on one leg and lift the other leg in front of you as you rotate into your rehab position. Then circle the leg three times clockwise and three times counterclockwise. Perform the same exercise with the leg to the side, and then finish with the leg behind you. Stand tall and lift out of your joints as you perform this drill.

While this exercise will help improve the mapping of the moving hip, it's the movement plan that sends reflexive stability signals to the opposite side, reinstating Agent M to her superhero status.

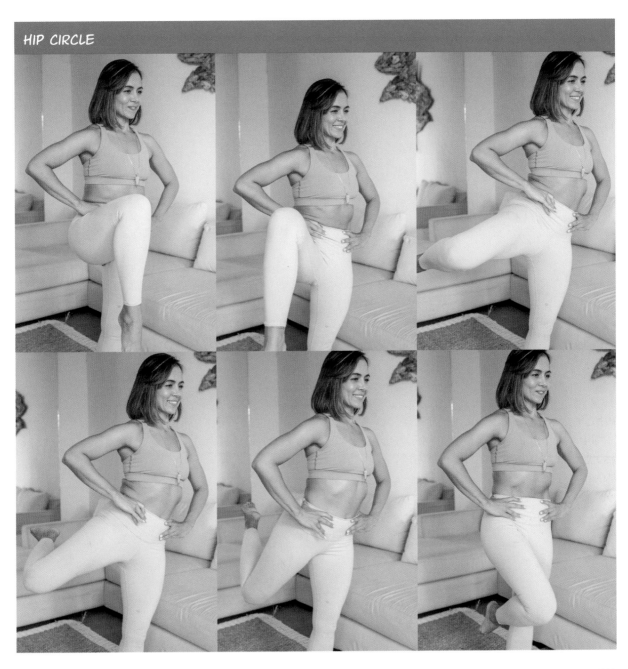

HIP CIRCLE

CHAPTER 8:

ELASTICATED LIMBS

Why have we placed your elasticated arms and legs in the same chapter? Although they are different limbs that have very different functional priorities, they share a lot of similarities.

The long arm bone (humerus) is basically a smaller version of the long leg bone (femur). The elbow and knee mimic each other (with a few little quirks that set them apart). There are two forearm bones (radius and ulna) and two lower leg bones (tibia and fibula). These bones link to the wrists and ankles, respectively, which are comprised of irregular-shaped bones, the carpals and tarsals. The hand has a few metacarpals, and the foot has metatarsals. Both finish with phalanges in the fingers and toes.[167]

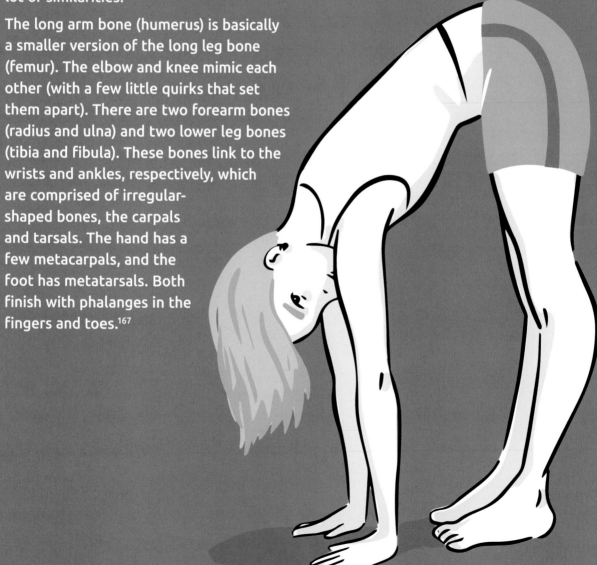

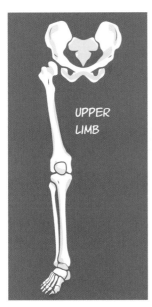

UPPER LIMB

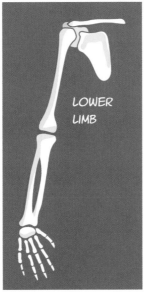

LOWER LIMB

The hands and feet occupy huge cortical real estate in the brain.[168,185] Therefore, improving their motor and sensory mapping can actually help improve the function of the body as a whole. The reason this is possible is because neurons that wire together fire together.[169] If we can light up massive parts of the brain before we hit the gym, dance floor, or yoga mat, our performance in our chosen movement discipline will be better.[168,170]

ELBOWS, KNEES, AND THE MARVELS OF TORQUE

If you look back at Body Map Man, you'll notice that elbows and knees are (or at least should be) in the stable camp. However, many self-respecting hypermobile people will happily whip out these joints and show off their extreme ranges, proving that stability is not the norm for these joints in our bendy bodies.[171]

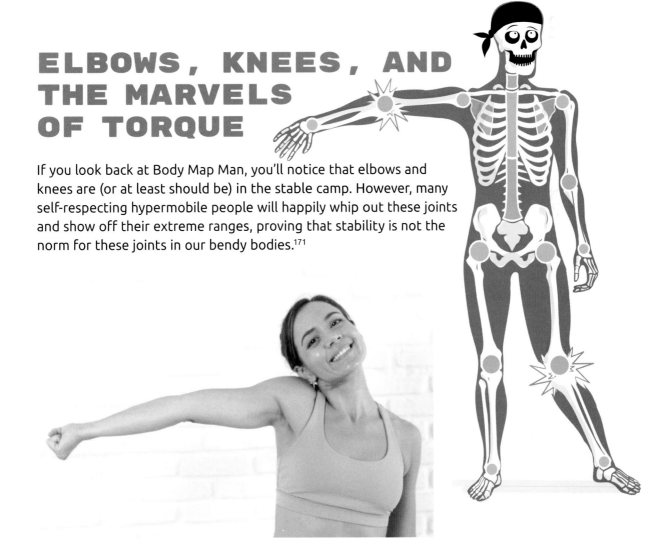

What can we do about this? Well, one piece of the puzzle is to make sure your proximal stability muscles are strong. Another strategy is to use torque.[172] **Forget twerking; we're into torquing.**

Way back in Chapter 3, which is all about the brain, we speak about using maximal tension to move through exercises to help improve mapping. Torque is one way to take this concept to the next level.

Torque is defined as a force being generated around an axis. It works for turning on your musculature when your limbs have multiple forces happening simultaneously.[173] For example, stand tall, keep your feet still, and then rotate your thighs outward. Now sustain this tension as you do a squat and notice how you can't just flop into your ligaments. Torque creates tension, aka *stability*.

Kelly Starrett, a CrossFit coach and physiotherapist, adapted this concept to help increase the strength generated around joints so that CrossFit athletes could lift much heavier weights safely.[174] We don't lift as heavy as CrossFit athletes do (massive presumption, we know, and a sincere apology if you're reading this and thinking, "Actually…"), but you can use this same concept whether you are doing yoga, resistance training, or even everyday movements like lifting your sleepy (and surprisingly heavy) three-year-old to bed.

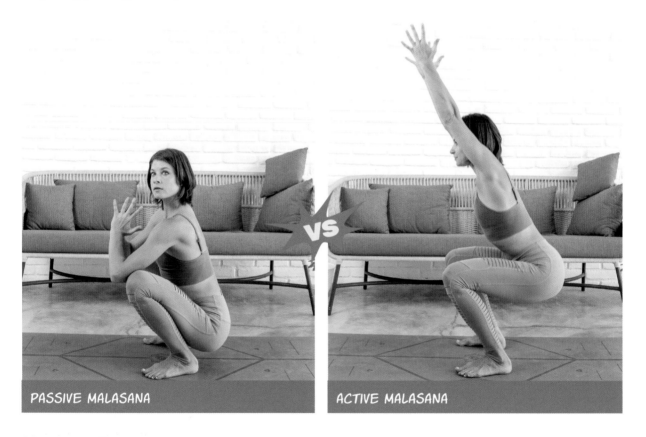

PASSIVE MALASANA — ACTIVE MALASANA

How to Torque

The long limb bone (humerus or femur) rotates either internally (toward the body) or externally (away from the body) depending on the desired action, while the hand or foot anchors the limb in the opposite direction.[173] For most hypermobile people, it's helpful to start off slowly, with the focus on externally rotating the long bone of the arm or leg and then anchoring the arm or foot with the index finger or big toe.

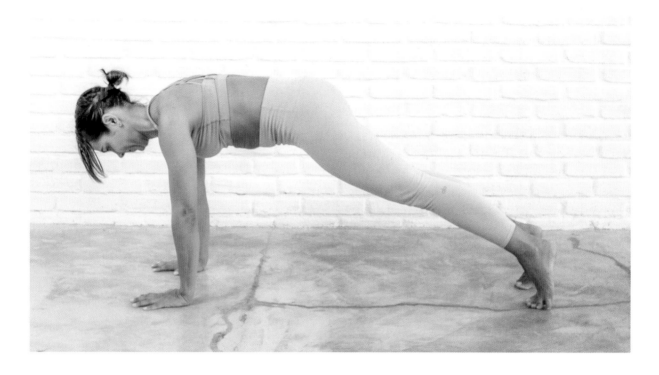

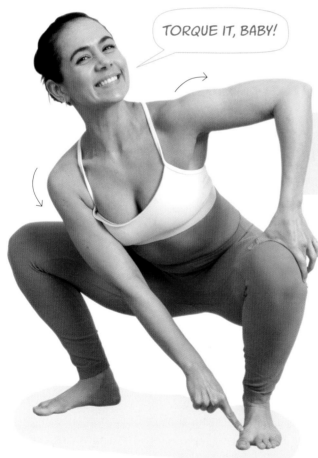

TORQUE IT, BABY!

In a squat, externally rotate your femurs while keeping your big toes grounded.

Please don't torque every minute of every day because doing so would just build unnecessary tension. Torque is a tool to use on occasion: if you're about to lift something really heavy, for example, or if you're working on improving your neural maps. (However, if you want to twerk every minute of every day, we have zero objections to that. Twerk to your heart's content.)

Elbow Stability

No doubt, one of the challenges we consistently see pop up in our Bendy Fam is how our elbows hyperextend, especially when bearing weight on our hands.

In this instance, healthy shoulder mechanics can make a positive difference, even though we're working on the efficiency of the elbow. As per usual, good ol' Serratus Shadow Wing Anterior is the hero we turn to. When you're bearing weight on your hands, the proximal stability the serratus provides helps prevent the elbow from collapsing into the ligaments.[175]

When we caution against hyperextending elbows and knees, we are highlighting the dangers of doing so *passively*. This is when the ligaments take the strain and their ability to provide stability is compromised. However, visibly hyperextending with your muscles ON is perfectly healthy and can help provide brain mapping for this additional range of motion.

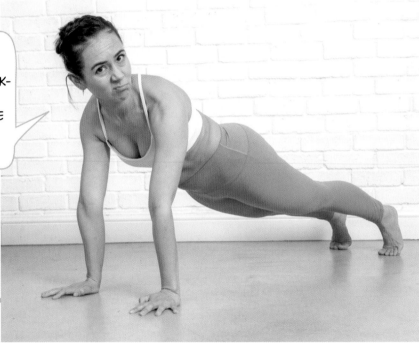

IF YOU'RE BEARING WEIGHT ON YOUR ARMS—FOR EXAMPLE, IN A PLANK—EXTERNALLY ROTATE YOUR UPPER ARMS WHILE KEEPING YOUR INDEX FINGERS DOWN.

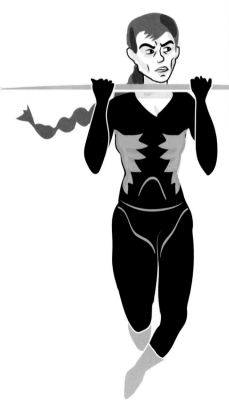

It's also always worth mixing up your training styles to challenge new muscles. For example, if your one true movement love is yoga and yoga alone, then bear in mind that it is a push-dominant discipline that predominantly uses your triceps. If your pull muscles (aka your biceps) aren't getting much opportunity to develop through exercises that involve pulling (for example, swimming, rowing, climbing, or resistance training), there will be a strength discrepancy around the elbow joint that might perpetuate the tendency to hyperextend.[177] Therefore, we will say it again: practice variety!

Elbow Circles

With your palm facing down, circle your forearm, from the elbow joint, inward toward your chest. Beyond the shoulder the circle continues, palm up. Repeat in the other direction.

Turn your palm up and circle outward toward your shoulder. As your hand approaches your shoulder, your palm will turn down to complete the circle.

ELBOW CIRCLES

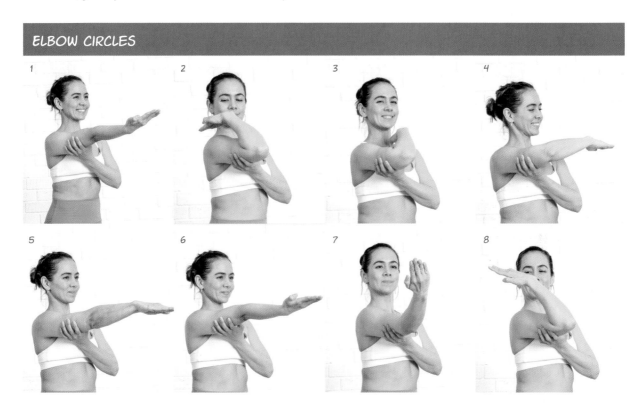

HYPEREXTENDED KNEES AND ELBOWS

Should we avoid hyperextension at all costs? The short answer is that it depends. Hyperextended or "locked" joints are not harmful if your myofascial system is supporting your ligaments. However, we hypermobile folks often collapse into joints such as elbows and knees, turning our muscles off and overstretching our ligaments. Our lack of proprioceptive awareness could lead to joint wear-and-tear down the line, so it's worth teaching the muscles to protect the joints into our fullest range of motion.[177] Therefore, don't be afraid of actively exploring hyperextension.

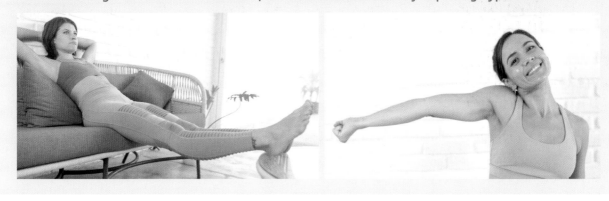

Knee Stability

Knees follow a similar story as elbows in that they also benefit from proximal stability, although their superhero is Sassy Stability Agent Gluteus Medius (see page 81). As we mentioned earlier, Agent M assists in keeping the knees out of a valgus position. We don't want you to think that valgus knees are all bad. Valgus is an important knee position that should be trained actively for side-to-side movements, such as for basketball or ice skating. Training the knee actively to tolerate all ranges is really important for its resilience and improved neural mapping.[177] What you want to avoid is flopping there unconsciously with every step you take.

Legs also want to make sure the balance of push and pull is adequate. Hamstrings are our pulling muscles that facilitate lifting heavy loads from a deadlift position, and quads are our pushing muscles that enable us to lift from a squat position. In some movement disciplines, we might favor one type over the other, which can lead to imbalances. For example, if on one side your hamstrings have never seen the weight of a shopping bag, and quadzilla has moved in on the other side, there is an increased chance your knees will hyperextend. Therefore, please mix it up (see page 114).

Knee Circles

Stand with a tall spine and your feet together and lock your knees actively. Move your knees to circle them in the same direction. Make the circle you create as big as possible, without moving your feet to compensate. Circle in both directions.

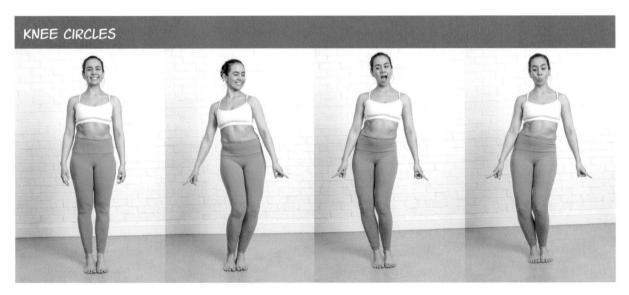

KNEE CIRCLES

Now have a go and circle one knee at a time with your legs wide apart. Step to the side with one leg bent and the other straight, and practice circling your knee in this new weighted position.

Next, it's time to add resistance. Either step into a booty band (a smaller circle) or if, you don't have one of those, use a double-looped resistance band. Shimmy the band over the tops of your knees and step to the side. With one leg straight and the other bent, circle the bent leg against the resistance of the band.

KNEE CIRCLES WITH RESISTANCE BAND

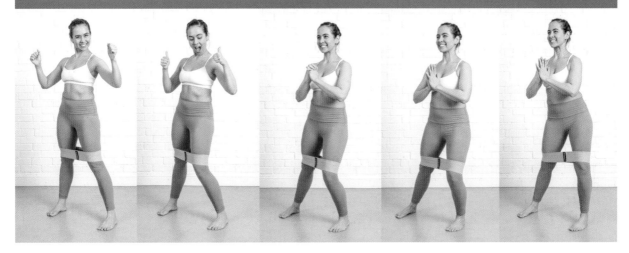

If you want to up the ante, slide the band down to your ankles and circle the leg there.

SINGLE-LEG KNEE CIRCLES

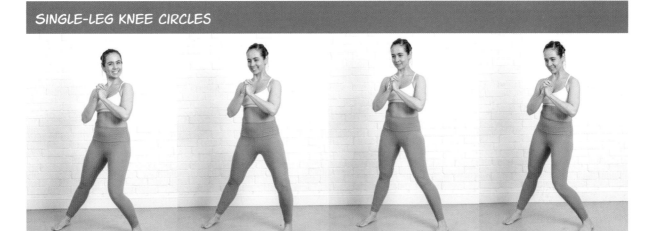

FOOT REST

This one isn't quite an exercise; it's more like a little word of warning. When your feet are resting on a foot stool, be mindful of your knees hyperextending passively. It's not uncommon for us to sit with our feet propped up, completely unaware, and when we stand up from that position, our knees ache. If you are going to take a load off, make sure your knees are supported.

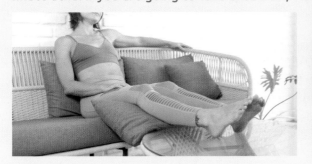
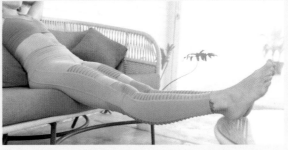

HANDS

Hands occupy a huge area of cortical real estate. (Remember the homunculus from page 40?) Not only do the hands take up a sizeable chunk of your movement cortex, but they also stretch over much of the sensory cortex.[178] Therefore, don't skip hand day! In addition to improving the dexterity of your hands, you can improve the sensory capacity of your hands by "washing" them before you train (see info box on page 131 for details on why).

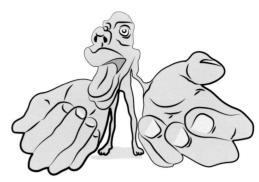

Stars

Close your fingers into a fist and reopen them as quickly as possible. Start with 30 repetitions and then build to 50.

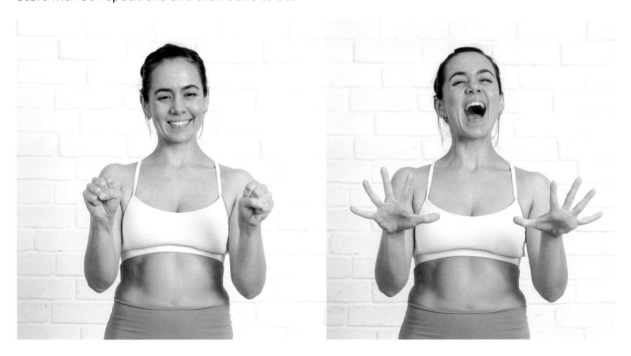

Finger Circles

Improving the dexterity of the individual joints is tricky at first, but you'll be surprised by how quickly you adapt and get the hang of it. See if you can circle the thumb three times clockwise and three times counterclockwise. Then progress through each individual finger, trying not to move the other fingers as you do. If this exercise is really challenging as first, and you have an easier time opening a beer can with your feet, use your opposite hand to hold the other fingers as the circling finger moves.

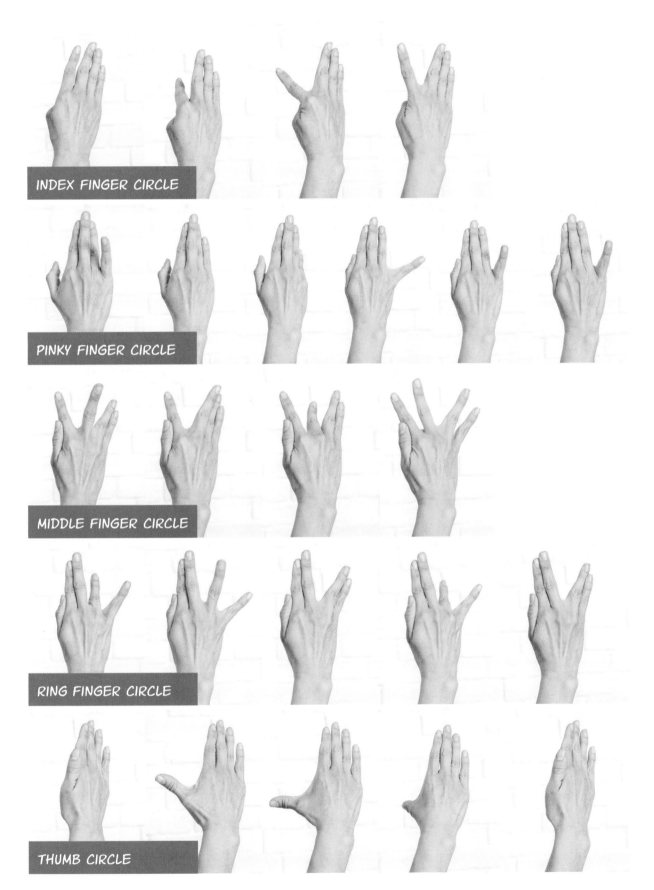

INDEX FINGER CIRCLE

PINKY FINGER CIRCLE

MIDDLE FINGER CIRCLE

RING FINGER CIRCLE

THUMB CIRCLE

Figure-Eights

Good old-fashioned wrist circles are fabulous, and we highly encourage their regular appearance in your workouts. But when wrist circles become too easy, the next step is to do figure-eights.

Start with your elbow bent 90 degrees with your palm facing up. Flex your wrist, imagining your palm high-fiving your bicep. Allow the little finger to lead the way as you turn your fingers down to the ground. Extend your wrist as if you were high-fiving another person. Again, little finger leads the way as your fingers rotate to point downward. Then repeat.

FIGURE-8 PALM UP

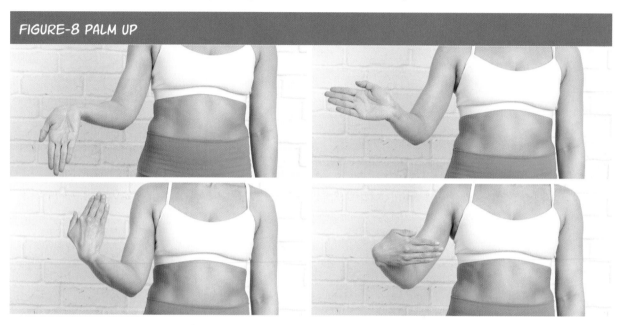

For the thumb to lead the way, begin with your palm facing down. Flex your wrist down toward your forearm so your fingers point down. Turn your hand with the thumb in the lead until your fingers point up. Extend your wrist until the palm is facing forward and your fingers point down. And finish the figure-eight with your thumb leading the way back to where you started.

FIGURE-8 PALM DOWN

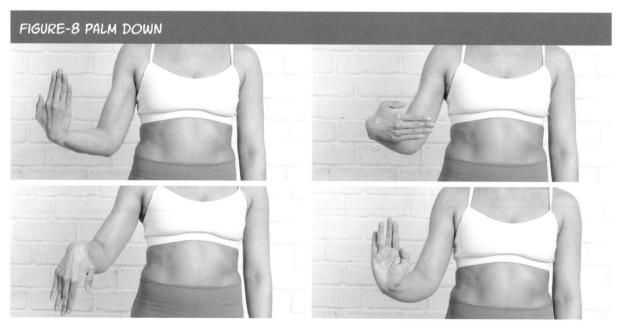

Wrist Glides

Bend your elbow 90 degrees and make a fist with your palm facing down. Keep your knuckles parallel to the floor as you glide your wrist from side to side. Then change the direction and glide the wrist up and down.

Now imagine your wrist hitting the four corners of a box—up, side, down, side. Eventually, smooth out the corners of the box and make a circle.

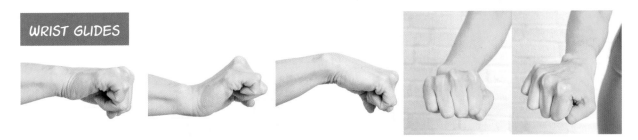

If you want to have strong wrists that would challenge the Hulk's, grab a resistance band and step one foot inside it. Hold the band in the hand on the same side and make a first. Practice the same progressions, starting with side-to-side and up-and-down; then make a box before trying smooth circles.

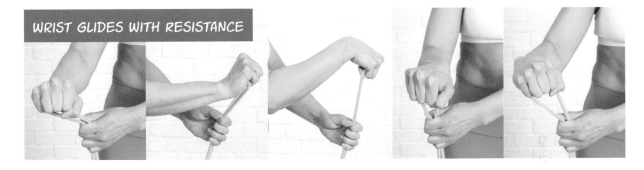

BRAIN FOOD AND BODY MASSAGE

The brain's main meal of choice is oxygen and glucose.[179] It draws these nutrients from the bottom of the brain upward and then consumes them from the back of the brain to the front.[180] When looking at how the brain is laid out, we notice that the sensory cortex gets the first shot of the incoming nutrients, before the motor cortex. To make use of this spongy soaking-up of energy, make sure you are breathing well, you have eaten enough, and you give yourself a good rub down before you train. It might seem silly at first, but lighting up your sensory cortex before you exercise actually improves your performance.

Massage your face, ears, and neck. Rub your shoulders and stroke your arms. "Wash" the palms and backs of the hands together. Try to reach your lower back and let your knuckles circle around your lower back and then rub your tummy. Stroke down the fronts of your legs and then up the backs. Finish with a foot massage.

All that should take just two to three minutes, and in the process you'll be lighting up your sensory cortex, which helps wake up your motor cortex.[181] Why? Because neurons that wire together fire together!

FEET

Before we share tips on how to tune up your tootsies, let's talk about shoes and convenience. Shoes are a wearable technology that weren't designed with your biomechanical interests at heart. Taller people with smaller feet were historically seen as sexier, so designers decided to capitalize on these insecurities. Shoes were created with heels for additional height and toe boxes that were small and curled up at the ends to make feet appear smaller. Early shoes also didn't take into consideration how many moving parts are in the feet or even what feet are functionally required to do each day. Instead, they froze feet into a single shape that is destined to walk short distances on unchallenging, flat surfaces.

Over time, these changes resulted in unfavorable adaptations. Every inch of increased heel height displaced the pelvis into an anterior tilt by 15 degrees.[182] The tiny toe boxes morphed the bone structure of feet and caused bunions. And the lack of movement over time severely weakened the musculature of the feet, negatively impacting the body as a whole.[122]

As muscles atrophied, bone density decreased, joints became deformed, ligaments were overstretched, proprioception in the feet was reduced, neural input started to wane, and even the brain's neuro-net changed in accordance with the lack of use.[183] That old saying "If you don't use it, you lose it" is 100 percent accurate, and it's observable in the entire population, not just in us flexies.

It doesn't stop there. Modern society decided to adapt the surfaces we walk on, making them even, flat, and unchallenging. As the years go by, our feet (and the corresponding brain tissues) become deconditioned, unsurprisingly making accidents especially prevalent among the elderly. The response to this problem has been to add more aids to facilitate balance, such as walking sticks and frames. In homes, we install walk-in showers and grab bars for the elderly to cling to. We fit chair lifts to conquer staircases and even sofas that, at the click of a button, automatically push a person to their feet without any need for muscular engagement—all in the name of helping people live longer. But these strategies are all Band-Aids, because they perpetuate the very reason they were needed in the first place and simultaneously hijack our quality of life. But why address the root cause of the problem when these sorts of aids can earn manufacturers huge sums of money?

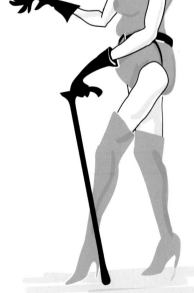

Modern life isn't a villain. It's just the result of humans collectively making life more convenient in the here-and-now, with some oversight about the importance of variety.

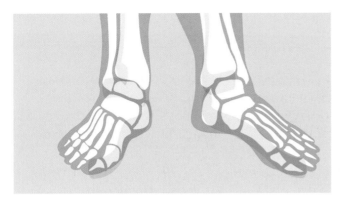

Our feet have 26 bones, 30 joints, and more than 100 muscles, tendons, and ligaments.[184] These intricate connections allow us to accommodate the endless variety found in nature. But without exposing our feet to these stressors, their capability to accommodate variety withers away.

Bendy Feet

Hypermobile people come in all shapes and sizes, but we all commonly adopt a habitual strategy to hang in our ligaments. The first most common strategy is flat arches, known as pronated feet. (Street lingo refers to them as "flat feet.") Another less-frequent strategy to avoid muscular engagement is when someone has high arches that collapse onto the outer ligaments, known as supination. Both of these strategies avoid using the myofascial system and instead rely on the ligamentous structure for support. While pronation and supination are normal foot positions required for healthy feet, we need to be alternating reflexively between both to harness their shock-absorbing superpowers.[184]

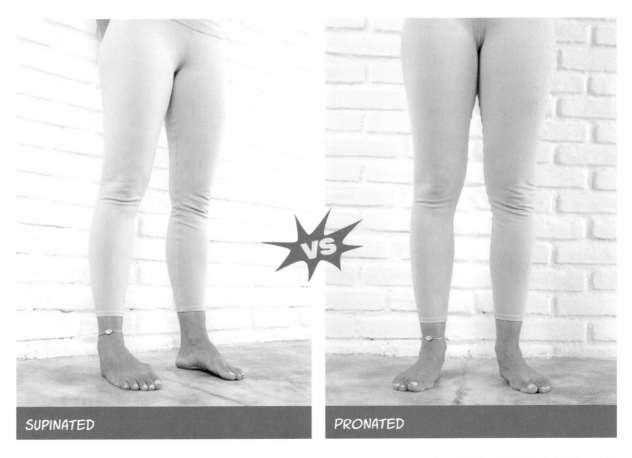

SUPINATED

PRONATED

Barefoot Shoes

Usually after learning about the detrimental effects of shoes, Bendies build a bonfire with the goal of destroying all their old shoes because they're keen to replace those instruments of torture with a set of barefoot shoes.

This is a worthy goal, but *be careful*! If you make the switch abruptly without having the right foundation, you might hurt yourself. Usually, we recommend three to six months of gradually easing into minimal shoes to make it sustainable and allow your tissues to adapt to the change in load. We also recommend making the switch to minimal footwear along with the following exercises, which will strengthen your feet so they become the foundation of a body that eats superpowers for breakfast.[122]

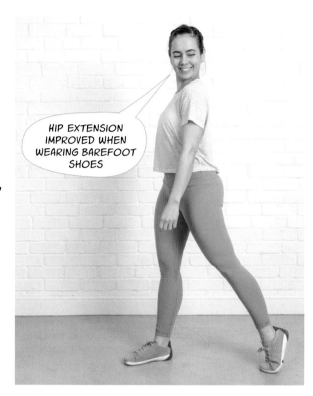

HIP EXTENSION IMPROVED WHEN WEARING BAREFOOT SHOES

Spiky Ball Rolls

If we had a magic wand, we would get everyone, everywhere walking barefoot outside. Since that trend is a little ways off, we recommend waking up the sensory maps of your brain with spiky balls. Roll your feet out for 20 to 30 seconds (or more if you like) daily, especially before your workout.

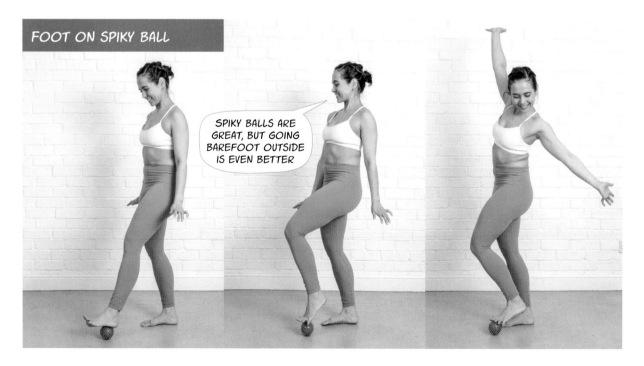

FOOT ON SPIKY BALL

SPIKY BALLS ARE GREAT, BUT GOING BAREFOOT OUTSIDE IS EVEN BETTER

Ankle Tilts Outer Foot

Loop a resistance band around the outside of your foot and pull on it with the opposite hand. Step the looped foot slightly forward on a diagonal and turn the foot in. Practice rolling onto the outer foot repeatedly. You can also turn the foot out or point it forward. In addition, practice moving the leg from the front diagonal position to the front, sides, and back diagonal to challenge how your foot experiences various directional forces.

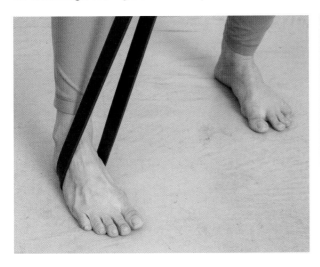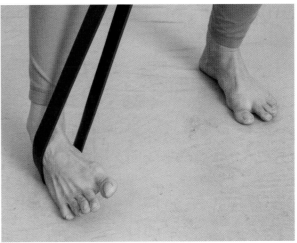

Ankle Tilts Inner Foot

Step into the band, holding the band in each hand. Take a big side step with your free foot and bend into that knee. Pull up hard against the band with the same hand as the bent knee to create resistance on the inner foot. Allow the foot inside the strap to roll repeatedly into the inner foot.

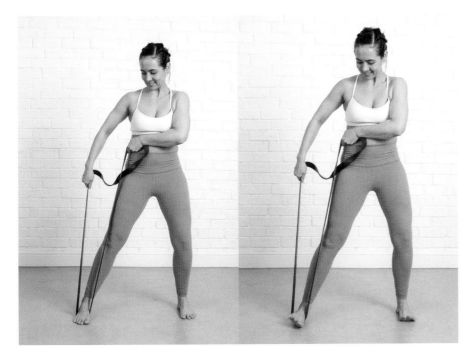

Ankle Tilts: In and Out

Step one foot into the band around the inner arch. Pull on both sides of the band for resistance and then tilt the foot from side to side.

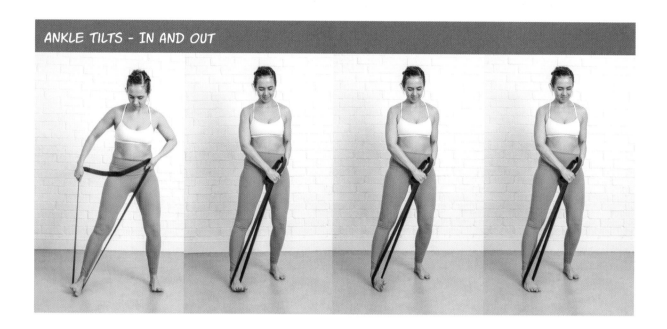

ANKLE TILTS – IN AND OUT

Foot Circles

Step one foot inside the band so it loops around the ball of your foot. Hold the band in each hand, like you're riding a horse. Practice circling your ankle against the resistance.

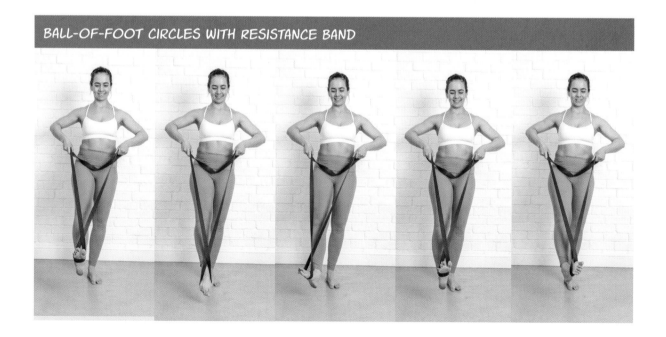

BALL-OF-FOOT CIRCLES WITH RESISTANCE BAND

Flexion Waves

Flex your foot and loop the band around the ball of your foot just under the toes. Curl your toes downward and allow the rest of the foot to follow, bit by bit. Once your foot is fully pointed, lift the toes and wave the foot back into the flexed position, bit by bit.

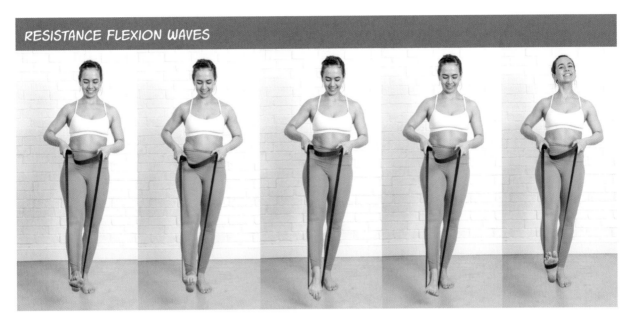

RESISTANCE FLEXION WAVES

Pointed-Toe Downdog

Come into a kneeling position with pointed toes. Place your hands on the floor, slowly push up into a pointed-toe downdog for a brief moment, and then lower back down. Allow your toes to push into the ground. If this position is uncomfortable, place a rolled-up towel under your feet.

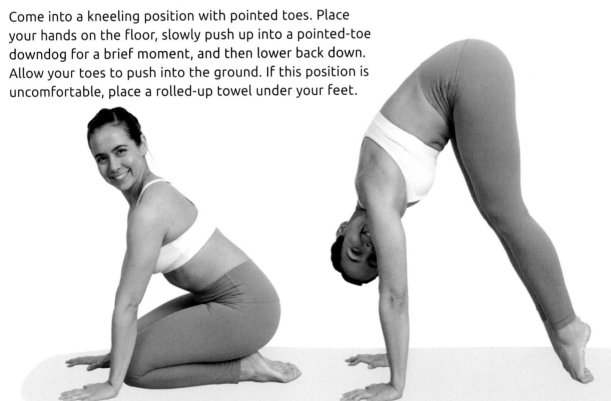

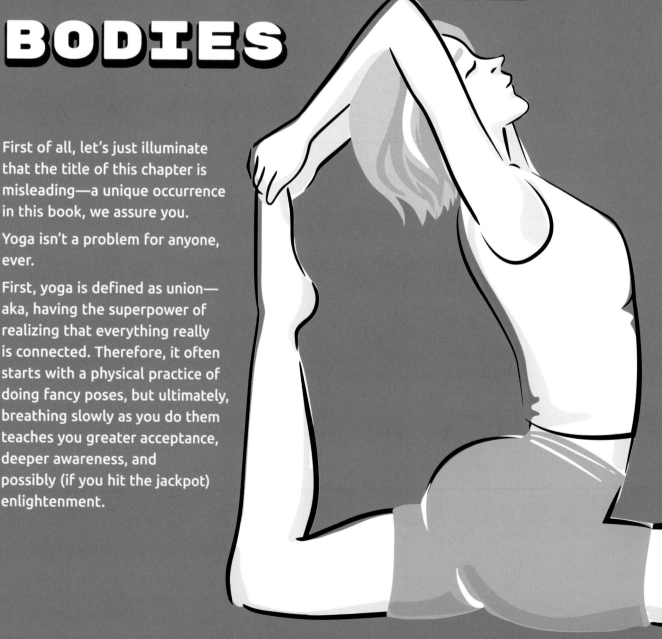

CHAPTER 9:

WHY YOGA IS A PROBLEM FOR HYPERMOBILE BODIES

First of all, let's just illuminate that the title of this chapter is misleading—a unique occurrence in this book, we assure you.

Yoga isn't a problem for anyone, ever.

First, yoga is defined as union—aka, having the superpower of realizing that everything really is connected. Therefore, it often starts with a physical practice of doing fancy poses, but ultimately, breathing slowly as you do them teaches you greater acceptance, deeper awareness, and possibly (if you hit the jackpot) enlightenment.

From the outside, yoga may look like a person sitting still with their eyes closed, chanting in a foreign language, and breathing in a way that looks like hyperventilating. Or, for a lot of people, yoga is about embodying their inner pretzel shape on a rectangular piece of rubber. Indeed, to an observer, it is impossible to know whether an inward journey is taking place. Only the practitioner knows for sure.

In this book, where we mention yoga, we are referencing the pretzel or postural element. In particular, we dive deep into the effects that those postures have on the typical human body and the alternate effects they have on a hypermobile body.

Before we get into that, we'd like to acknowledge that a deeper, inward journey is available with everything in life, not just meditating, chanting, breathing, or busting shapes on a rubber mat. Reading a book can be your yoga *(svadhyaya)*. In the same way, surfing, gardening, lifting weights, or eating a juicy pear one slow, mindful, gratitude-filled bite at a time can be yoga. If the practitioner is experiencing some form of connection of mind, body, breath, and self, and if the practitioner leaves the experience with a deeper awareness of their infinitesimally brief yet simultaneously eternal significance in the grander timeline of existence, then it could be argued that what is happening is yoga. Amen!

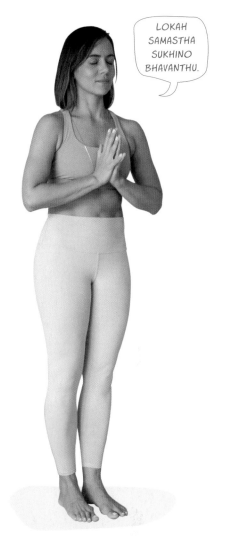

LOKAH SAMASTHA SUKHINO BHAVANTHU.

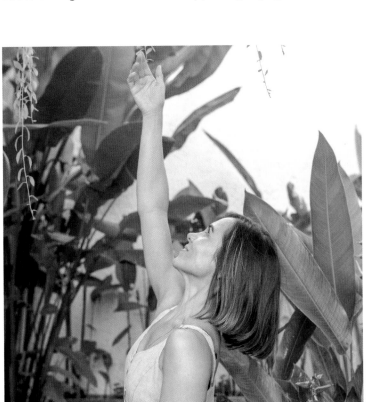

Some may disagree. But even the fact that there is disagreement is testament to the esoteric and deeply personal nature of the journey that is yoga.

And so, on that note, lapping up the information from this book will not only change (or—fingers crossed, with all stability muscles turned on—already has changed!) how you move on your yoga mat and how you hold your body upright in everyday life, but also take you deeper into understanding your intention behind why and how you move. Now that's *yoga!*

IS YOUR EGO HYPERMOBILE?

We talk about curbing our flexibility. Well, how about curbing your ego?

We believe, and we hope that by now you also believe, that hypermobility basically makes you superhuman!

Because of our tendency toward bendiness, there are a lot of things we find easy that our hypomobile comrades work on for months or even years.

But being able to do things with your body isn't really what makes a person superhuman. Maybe that's true in the sports world where physical feats are rewarded no matter the athlete's attitude, but in the real world, and certainly in the yoga world, it's never really about the shapes you can make with your body. All of our favorite superheroes are more than their superpowers. It's what they *do* with their superpowers.

Yes, we need to build strength into our floppy bodies. On top of that, we may face a harder lesson in humility than many of our hypomobile comrades do—at least when it comes to holding back in asanas that we know we can push ourselves into, even if it's painful.

We're talking about the ego, hypermobility, and learning a superhuman level of humility.

It has often been suggested that the number one cause of injury in yoga—for bendies and non-bendies alike—is the ego.[186] And your loving authors will be the first to admit that our egos have been the biggest hurdle we've faced when it comes to amending our practice to care for our hypermobile joints.[187]

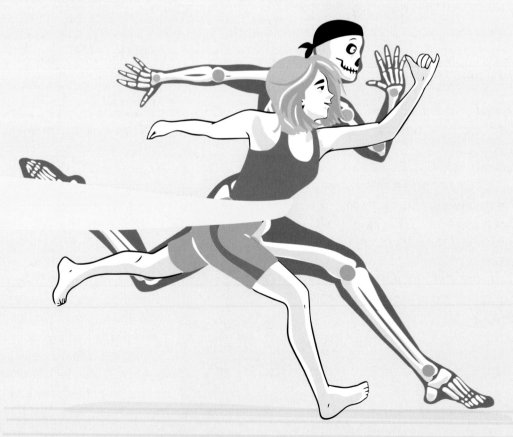

ADELL'S STORY

There's a yoga class near where I live that I used to love taking because it was very, very challenging, and I love a challenge. As I went through the class, I could see in my peripheral vision my fellow students nailing postures that most yoga teachers wouldn't attempt. They're often postures that I can do, too, but they hurt my shoulders and low back, so I modify them.

I could almost hear my ego whimpering and squirming with discomfort as I held back and didn't go as deep, using my strength and not relying on gravity to pull me into a pose.

But then it would happen—the teacher would get to the peak pose, my ego was bruised and battered from a whole class of holding back, and all the students around me were struggling with the peak pose. It would be one I could do easily if I dumped into my low back, which I knew could leave me with a backache for the rest of the day and possibly do further damage long term.

But my ego would say, "It's now or never!" and before I knew it, I'd be smugly moving into a ridiculous backbend that served no purpose. But ahhh, that feeling when you know you're the only one in the room who can do something—when the teacher says, "Great job, Adell," or even, "Everyone watch how Adell does it."

Every time, I would give myself a little talking-to as I gripped my back like I was auditioning for a painkiller commercial. I'd say, "You know better than that, Adell. Why did you do it?" Whereas other people were getting closer to their goals of getting the splits or grabbing their foot in dancer pose, I was slowly working toward my goal of prioritizing my body's needs over my ego's desires. In each session, I got a little closer, until one day I finally walked out of that class EXHAUSTED from staying out of end range and also feeling zero pretzel FOMO.

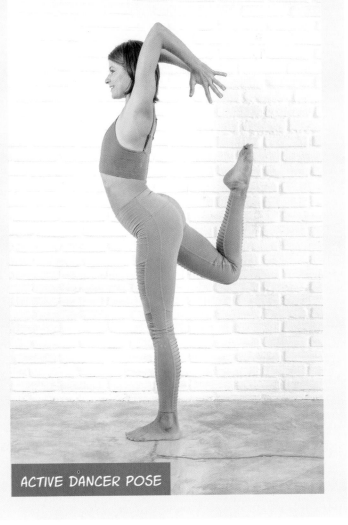

ACTIVE DANCER POSE

CELEST'S STORY

I became a yoga teacher, and soon after starting, I was teaching so many classes that I hit burnout. I decided then that the only way out was to grow my brand and business so that I could negotiate better pay and eventually cut back on the crazy hours I was working. To do so, I turned my attention to Instagram, desperate to grow my following to help me step off the hamster wheel.

Always one who likes to do my homework, I researched the best accounts and realized that the key to growth was bending in ways few other people could bend. I remember those cold December days when I would head out in yoga leggings and a crop top with a photographer to bend over backward, ignoring the pain from the cold and the discomfort in my joints, in the hope that my account would grow. I realize that this was desperation fueled by my ego's desire for validation. I kept thinking, "Why would anyone like a picture of me doing downward dog?"

When my body had had enough and I could no longer afford regular physiotherapy, I decided it was time to change my strategy. I began to look at my account as a way to educate rather than as a way to impress people. I started refining my knowledge and applied the principles I was learning. The incredible transformation I could feel in my body and see in the bodies of my students was far more compelling than the need to grow my 'gram. I'm so grateful my body sang signals of pain and discomfort, warning me to get out of the stupid coal mine my ego had created.

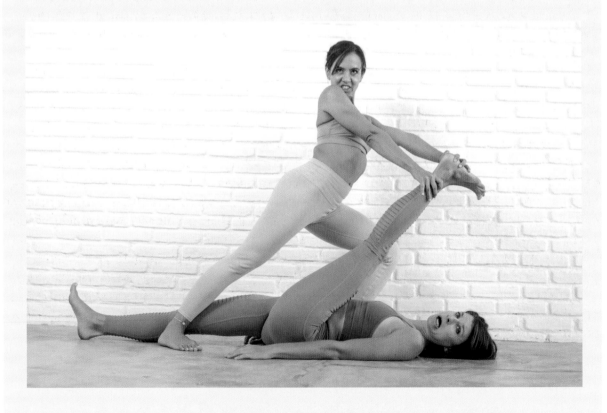

It's like a drug. You know it's bad for you, but you can't stop yourself. And then, after the high has worn off, you remember why you said you'd never do it again.

Humility. That's the real yoga.

Here's the thing: if you have more work to do to learn humility than the average person, then the end result is that you've had a longer, greater, more powerful lesson than someone who didn't need as much.

So we hypermobile people may not need to do much training for flexibility. We've already reached other people's flexibility goals. But perhaps where we can hone our superpower is in our journey toward being humble yoga practitioners.

Take this book not only as a volcanic eruption of information on anatomy and biomechanics, but also as a guide for refining your ability to notice, listen, and accept. Allow the issues raised and questions posed to heighten your perception of the world as the entirely subjective experience that it is. Peel your mind open to the possibility that each and every minute of your life can be perceived in an infinite number of ways. The only person responsible for deciding on which way it's perceived is *you*.

So, with that said, what this chapter *should* be called is

Why Modern Postural Yoga Asana the Way It Is Taught in Many (but Certainly Not All) Yoga Studios Is a Problem for Hypermobile Bodies

Whatever your belief about what yoga is or is not, it's generally agreed that many of the postures done in a typical yoga class came from India, although the majority of them originated not so long ago. While fifteen postures are listed in the ancient text of the Hatha Yoga Pradipika, most postures that are thought of as "traditional" and are referred to with Sanskrit names were born out of a mixture of Swedish gymnastics and Indian bodybuilding and made their way into the practice of yoga in the early to mid twentieth century.[188,228]

On the surface, yoga looks old, and therefore it has to be the best thing since sliced bread, right? Doesn't older equal better? Well, it's worth mentioning that around the same time in history when these postures were making their way into the practice of yoga, many prominent Western doctors believed that lobotomies were the best treatment for mental health disorders.[229] Also, the Indian patriarchs who practiced these postures lived in considerably different ways than twenty-first-century Westerners (and a lot of Easterners, for that matter), and unfortunately, a lot of what we've inherited in modern postural yoga was suitable for the people who created it but is less suitable for us. But yoga went viral, making its way off the shores of India, eventually mooring on the shores of the West and later the rest of the world. With all of this said, we should shift our focus to our evolutionary needs and away from what gurus think is cool.

Just as asana (poses) has evolved from the time of Krishnamacharya (an old yoga dude), begetting Iyengar and Ashtanga (other forms of shapey yoga), which begot Rocket, Dharma Yoga, Vinyasa (modern, shapey yoga), and a multitude of other styles, asana will continue to evolve. We hope that this book might be a part of the evolution of yoga asana into an entirely (as opposed to occasionally) intelligent movement practice that ensures the longevity of all bodies.

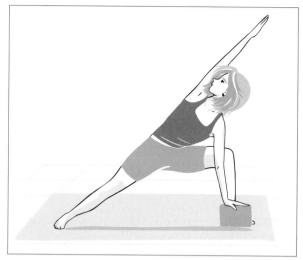

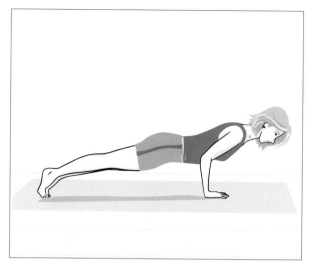

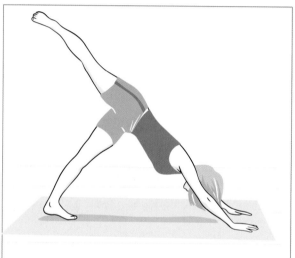

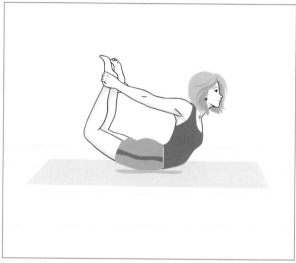

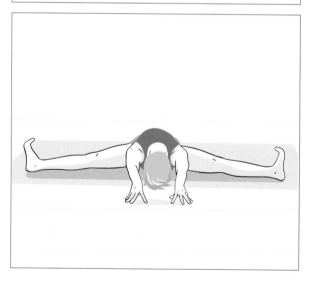

Because right now, sadly it's not.

Yoga can cause serious injury in more ways than one. Pushing beyond the natural range of motion, repeatedly practicing the same imbalance-causing sequences,* and failing to consider the postural weaknesses created by our modern lifestyles of sitting in chairs and having our phones do everything for us are just three ways that yoga is painting itself as a villain to the health of our bodies.[108,189] Some of these injuries are even named after their most common victims: "yoga butt," "yoga shoulder," and "Ashtangi knees."

---

*Have we mentioned that most traditional yoga classes favor hamstring stretches over hamstring strengtheners and internal shoulder rotations over external shoulder rotations and offer only pushing and no pulling?

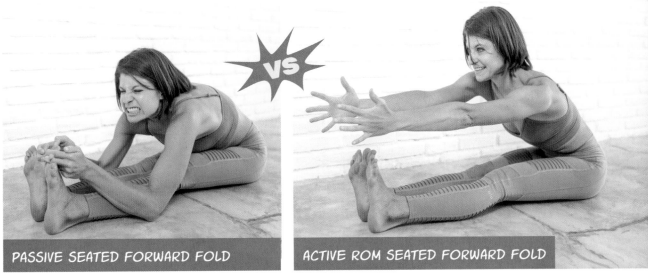

PASSIVE SEATED FORWARD FOLD   ACTIVE ROM SEATED FORWARD FOLD

Okay, maybe we just made up "Ashtangi knees," but that's because Adell once went to a weekend of workshops with a prominent Ashtanga teacher. For sale at the back were little cushions about the size of a rolled-up washcloth. When she asked what they were for, she was told that they were meant to be placed behind the knee in postures where the knee bends to the point of causing pain. The cushions helped alleviate that pain.

How about avoiding what causes the pain in the first place so you don't need to buy little cushions? Doesn't that make more sense?

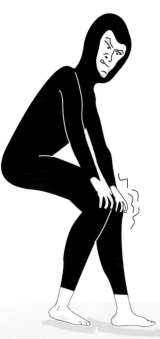

A NOTE ON INJURIES

We view injuries in much the same way that we view heartbreak—as something that hurts like hell and that we attempt to avoid at all costs. However, it will most likely happen to all of us at some point in life, and injuries can teach us a whole lot about ourselves and allow us to feel more empathy and compassion for others. Getting injured is also a beautiful and wonderful sign that we at least tried, experienced, *lived* something...even if it didn't turn out the way we hoped.

Let your injuries be your yoga. Allow them to be opportunities to learn about yourself. Take that learning and apply it *to ensure injuries don't happen again!* Especially since injuries in yoga are avoidable.

Let's leave the injuries to the extreme sports fanatics and freak accidents from now on, shall we?

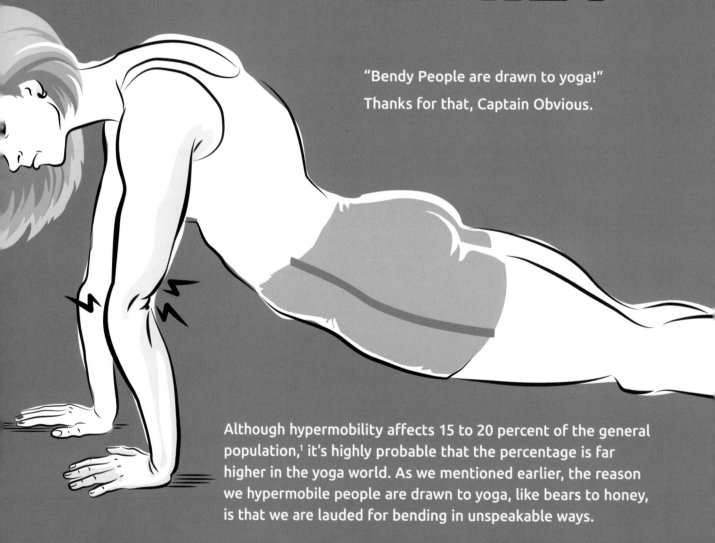

CHAPTER 10:

THE BENDY PERSON'S YOGA SURVIVAL KIT

"Bendy People are drawn to yoga!"
Thanks for that, Captain Obvious.

Although hypermobility affects 15 to 20 percent of the general population,[1] it's highly probable that the percentage is far higher in the yoga world. As we mentioned earlier, the reason we hypermobile people are drawn to yoga, like bears to honey, is that we are lauded for bending in unspeakable ways.

However, another reason we Bendies find ourselves reappearing like Houdini on the mat, come rain or shine, is that yoga provides *anxiety pacification tools* that other movement disciplines simply don't.[190] Best of all, we don't get weird and confused looks from people when we say things like, "I'm just a highly sensitive person. I feel *everything*." (Yeah, FYI, that's not ESP, it's JHS.)

We hope by now we've infiltrated your psyche so that the rest of this paragraph seems like the most mind-numbingly obvious thing ever: traditional yoga asana has an imbalanced ratio of flexibility training to strength training.[190] *All hail the stretching, and speak not of any strength except that of your ujjayi breath.*[191] As a result, it's not surprising that many doctors, physiotherapists, and osteopaths, as well as other healthcare professionals, advise their hypermobile patients to avoid yoga or preferably run away screaming bloody murder.

Herein lies the stark dilemma: do we keep going to yoga and risk hurting our wet noodle bodies, or do we ditch it for lifting weights and sacrifice our mental health?

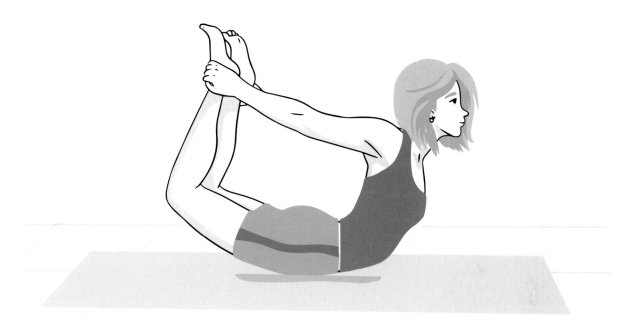

KNOWLEDGE BOMB!

HERE'S THAT IMPORTANT INFORMATION AGAIN: YOU CAN CONTINUE PRACTICING YOGA IF YOU ARE HYPERMOBILE. YOU JUST NEED TO MODIFY CORRECTLY.

BOOM

Yoga, dance, gymnastics, Pilates, CrossFit, underwater hockey, toe wrestling, extreme ironing, and plucking a banjo are all things you can continue doing (or pick up) if you're hypermobile. These activities are also ticking time bombs for injury if not done with stability. We suggest you drool over the biomechanics and drills sections of this book regularly to help keep yourself on the straight and narrow.

For the purposes of this chapter, let's focus on yoga and how you can modify your practice to ensure you stay safe.

YOGA CUES TO BE WARY OF

Here's a quick index of some yoga things that we have already discussed in their relevant biomechanics chapters. Turn back to those chapters if you want more information on these particular cues.

When we discussed binding your arms in Chapter 7, we mentioned how we spend a disproportionate amount of time in internal versus external rotation. That's fine, because we do more internal rotation in everyday life anyway. *However,* when we bind, we are opening every door and window for Passive Range of Misery Man to make himself at home in our shoulder joints. So, when binding, try to do it without clasping your hands or touching your arms to other body parts.

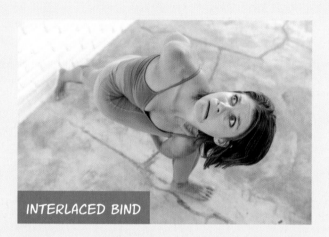

INTERLACED BIND

When we talked about relaxing your glutes in your backbend in Chapter 6, we detailed why "relax your glutes" is not a cue that should go with any backbending posture.

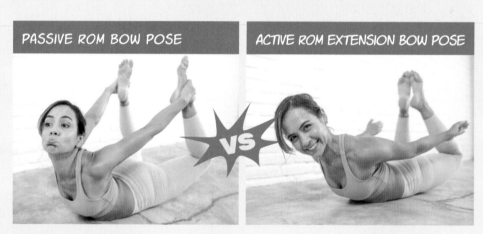

PASSIVE ROM BOW POSE

ACTIVE ROM EXTENSION BOW POSE

VS

When it comes to downward-facing dog:

- The cue "Draw your shoulders down away from your ears" should be ignored by yoga practitioners and never uttered again by yoga teachers when the arms are overhead. Flip back to Chapter 7 for more on this.

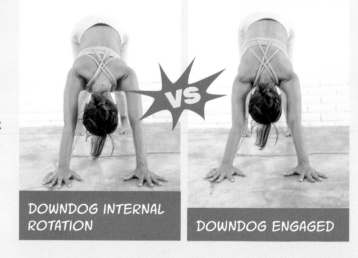

DOWNDOG INTERNAL ROTATION

DOWNDOG ENGAGED

VS

- In Chapter 8, under "How to Torque," we mentioned pressing your heels into the floor to help describe the ideal way the feet move in relation to the ankles. You want stability in the feet and mobility in the ankles. But a lot of Bendies have collapsed arches that do all the moving when yoga instructors encourage pressing the heels down (instead of the ankles) in downward dog. Encouraging a nice footprint with arches lifting away from the floor may help you avoid sad and collapsed feet.

Hero pose and lotus pose are two postures that can be deadly for the knees. Remember Body Map Man in Chapter 2 and how he shows us that the knees are where we ought to be stable? And AROM the Protector would beg that you keep your knees stable by moving into postures with muscular control through the joints. If you look at these poses, you'll likely see why we consider them to be in Passive Range of Misery Man's territory.

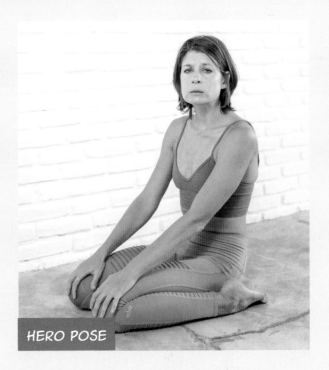

HERO POSE

- Hero pose uses gravity to passively pull the knees into extreme flexion. We recommend replacing this posture with mini "sissy squats" to build strength in your quads and glutes. For sissy squats, you bend only in the knees and ankles, lift your heels from the floor as you lean back, bend your knees, and keep your hips straight.

- You likely get into lotus pose by using your hands to pull your ankles over your thighs. Then, with your legs in this knot, you need zero activation to keep yourself there. This means the ligaments in your knees could be at great risk of being overstretched. We recommend replacing lotus with cobbler pose and pressing the outsides of your feet into your mat to keep your legs active. BONUS: Try pressing the soles of your feet together and lifting them off the mat without leaning your chest back!

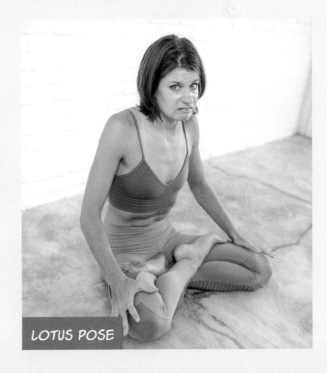

LOTUS POSE

DON'T GO TO END RANGE OF MOTION

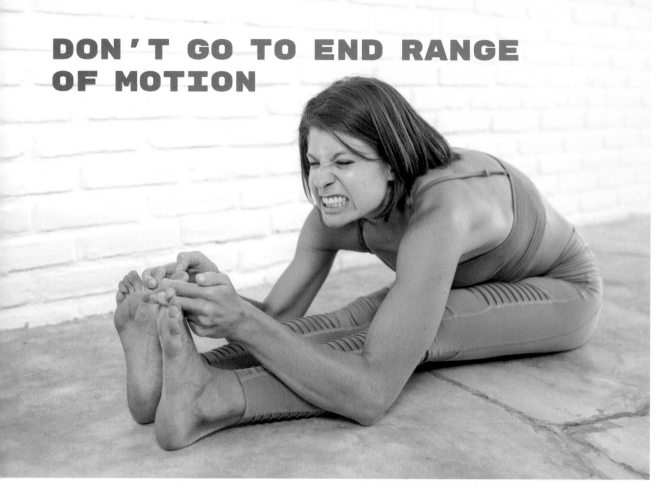

You may remember from Chapter 1 that our bodies have different ranges of motions and barriers in place, put in place by the nervous system to keep us safe. Just to recap, these barriers are mostly neurological, but there are also elements of restriction that are myofascial (in the muscles and fascia) and skeletal (in the bones).

- The range of motion that is *active* is generally safe, thanks to the strong arms of AROM the Protector (**swoon**). We can put our bodies there mindfully, with control, and hold them in place, maybe even against resistance such as gravity or weight.

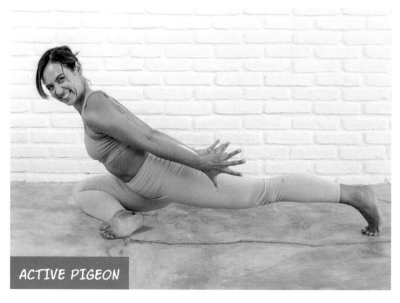

ACTIVE PIGEON

- Our *passive* range of motion begins when we need some sort of outside force to move a body part farther than we can get it using our active range of motion.

- *End range* of motion, also known as the anatomical barrier, is a way to explain the point past which your body physically will not go without sustaining damage.

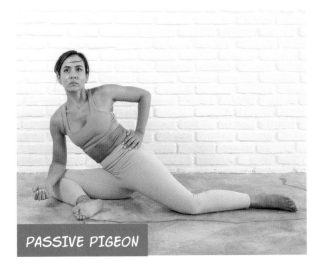

PASSIVE PIGEON

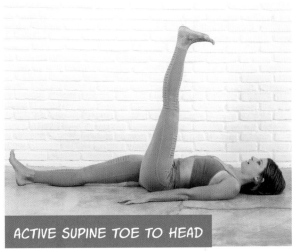

ACTIVE SUPINE TOE TO HEAD

Guess where hypermobile people tend to go when they stretch? End range. Guess what a lot of yoga cues encourage, either intentionally or unintentionally? Going to end range. And guess what happens at end range? Stretching that-which-should-not-be-stretched causes serious and sometimes irreparable damage to ligaments. (Think back to the sticky tack example from page 31.)

Understanding the difference between active range of motion (AROM) and passive range of motion (PROM) will keep you safe in all movement practices. If you want to go to "end" range, make sure it's the end of your active range of motion and not all the way to the anatomical barrier.

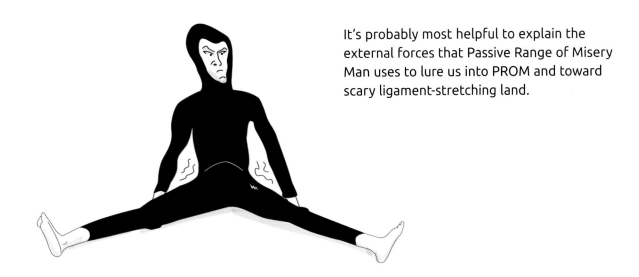

It's probably most helpful to explain the external forces that Passive Range of Misery Man uses to lure us into PROM and toward scary ligament-stretching land.

Hands and Other Body Parts

They may be your own hands or the hands of someone helping you stretch or "go deeper," such as a yoga teacher. It could also be another body part: think of using your elbow on the outside of the opposite knee in a twisting lunge or a twisting chair pose. A third example is the connection between the foot and thigh when a yogi's legs are in lotus pose. Cues that encourage this type of passive movement are the first ones to be wary of. You may hear phrases like the following in a lot of yoga classes:

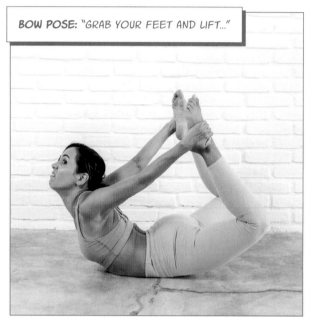

BOW POSE: "GRAB YOUR FEET AND LIFT..."

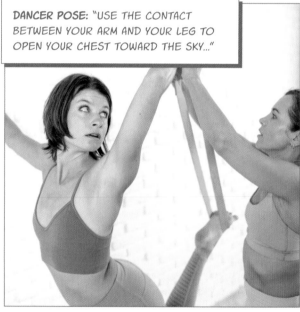

DANCER POSE: "USE THE CONTACT BETWEEN YOUR ARM AND YOUR LEG TO OPEN YOUR CHEST TOWARD THE SKY..."

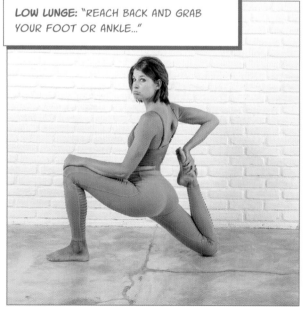

LOW LUNGE: "REACH BACK AND GRAB YOUR FOOT OR ANKLE..."

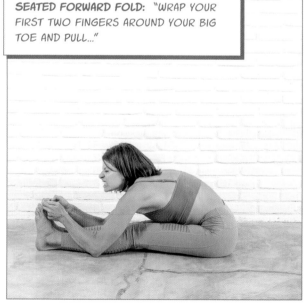

SEATED FORWARD FOLD: "WRAP YOUR FIRST TWO FINGERS AROUND YOUR BIG TOE AND PULL..."

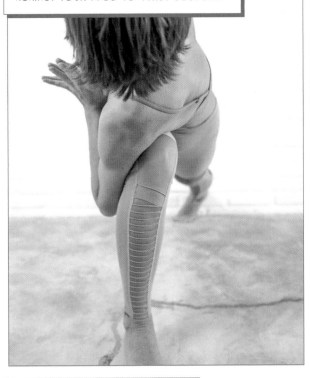

While the body parts doing the pulling or pushing are active (yay!), other areas are completely passive. For example:

BOW POSE: WITH HANDS HOLDING THE FEET, THE POSTERIOR CHAIN CAN BE INACTIVE, POSSIBLY LEADING TO A CRUNCHED LOW BACK.

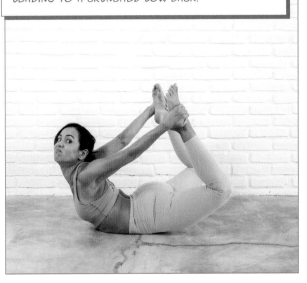

LOW LUNGE: WHEN YOUR HAND IS PULLING YOUR FOOT TO YOUR BUTT, YOUR HAMSTRINGS AND GLUTES MISS OUT ON AN AWESOME WORKOUT.

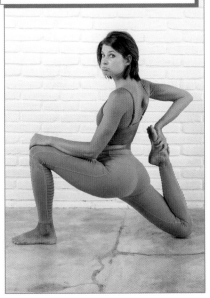

TWISTED LUNGE: LETTING PRESSURE BETWEEN THE ELBOW AND THE KNEE PRODUCE YOUR TWIST MEANS YOUR OBLIQUES AND INTERCOSTAL MUSCLES CAN SNOOZE AND YOUR INNER ELASTIDOG (NERVOUS SYSTEM) DOESN'T LEARN COOL THORACIC ROTATION TRICKS.

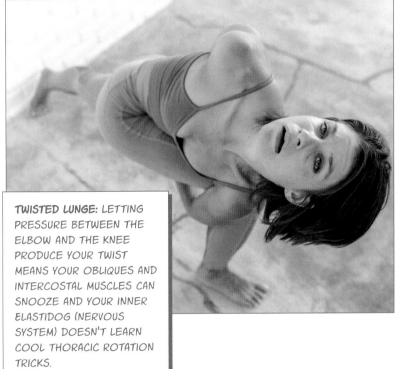

Consider for a moment what it would look like to do the previous list of postures without letting your hands or arms touch your legs or feet—or put this book down and try it right now! Instead, try these types of poses using these Bendy suggestions:

- Do the movement without making contact between the two body parts. (You can fake it if you don't want to be that person in class doing their own thing. Or go rogue and be that person. We're rooting for you!)

- If you must make contact, move into these postures as much as possible with the help of AROM the Protector and keep all those muscles active instead of letting the pulling, pushing, and pressing coax you into relaxation.

- If someone else is pushing or pulling you deeper, ask them to back off. Explain that you want to work on strength and you're not interested in going deep into postures.

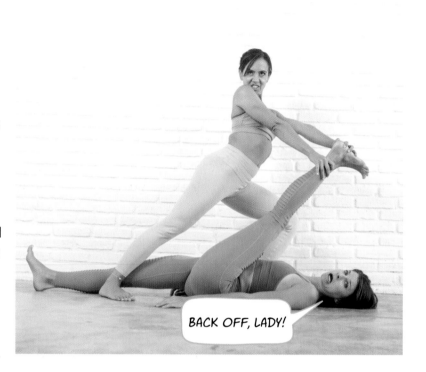

Gravity

Depending on the orientation of your body in a particular yoga posture, gravity may be a force of resistance that you have to work against, or it may be a force that contributes to you sinking toward your end range of motion.

Remember, whatever shape you make and wherever you are in space, gravity is always pulling in the same direction—toward the Earth's core. It's what makes holding plank position or raising your leg in front of you so difficult. So working against gravity can be a great way to build strength. But in some postures, gravity can be a force for Passive Range of Misery Man—unless you resist Earth's pull.

Watch out for these common postures where gravity can make it all too easy to be sucked into Misery Man's lair:

- **Anjanayasana (low lunge):** Letting your hips sink downward, and perhaps letting the arch of your front foot collapse, allowing your front knee to fall inward, too, is a recipe for disaster.

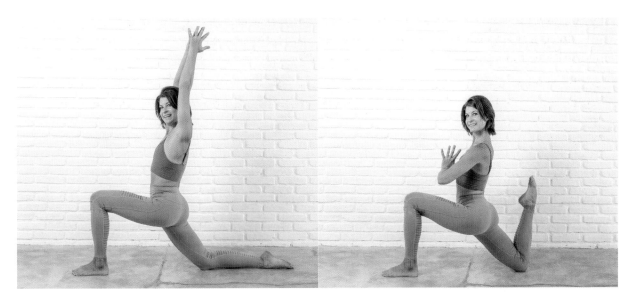

– *Instead:* Lift your hips up away from gravity, staying just outside that end range of motion by squeezing your thighs together, keeping the arches of your feet active, and ensuring that your front knee stays in line with your ankle. (It is not important to have the knee stacked over the ankle.)

– *Optional:* Pull your back heel toward your butt using just the strength of your hamstrings and glutes.

• **Paschimottanasana (seated forward bend):** Slumping your chest over your thighs with your legs and core relaxed could be a chance for your hamstrings to get overstretched.

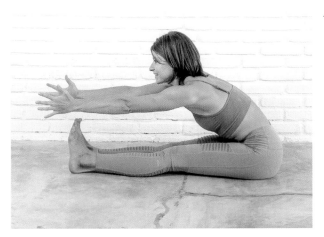

– *Instead:* Press your heels into the floor and pull your toes toward your face to activate your leg muscles, keeping some space between your torso and legs.

• **Ustrasana (camel pose):** Flopping backward, usually at the expense of your lower back, puts you at risk of succumbing to gravity and potentially to injury.

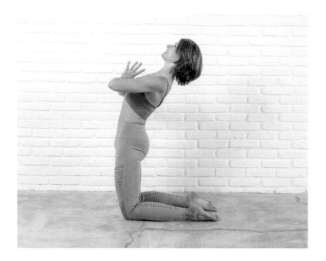

– *Instead:* A good way to understand where you can move actively and where gravity begins to take control is to lower only to a point from which you can lift yourself back up. Remember, however, what we covered on page 35 with Body Map Man, and how the lumbar spine needs to be stable. So spread the bend by extending in your hips and thoracic spine, and avoid doing all the bending from your lower back.

Momentum

For the purposes of this chapter, think of moving with momentum being the opposite of moving with control. We use momentum when we jump, leap, fling, or kick ourselves through a movement or transition. When you move with control, you could pause at any point along the way from one posture to the next and hold yourself statically. When you remove control and replace it with momentum, there ain't no stoppin' that runaway train. In many cases, moving with momentum means that movements require less effort than if you slowed them down and moved with control.

Let's try a common yoga transition as an example. From one-legged downward-facing dog, step the elevated foot forward, placing it between your hands, and lift your chest up to a lunge.

Seems easy, but actually it's mega tough. This is one of those transitions that make yoga newbies say, "I didn't know yoga was gonna kick my butt!" One way to make it less butt-kicking is to use momentum to fling the leg forward. Try moving through this transition so slowly that at every point along the way, you can pause and hold your leg up in space. You'll probably be saying, "Okay, okay, I get it! I know the difference now between control and momentum!"

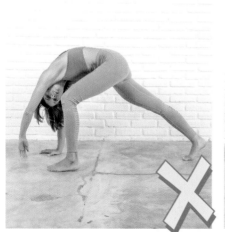

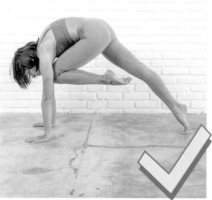

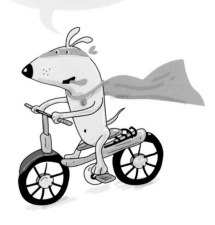

"IT'S EASIER WHEN I GO FASTER!"

Bendy People are especially adept at relying on momentum to compensate for a lack of strength to move from one point to another.

Another place where controlled movement commonly gets really shy is moving out of a posture that involves holding a leg up. For example, if you're using your hand to hold your foot to your butt in a low lunge, can you lower the leg slowly back to your mat when you release it? Can you fight the flop?

Try these Bendy suggestions for dealing with momentum:

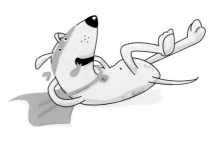

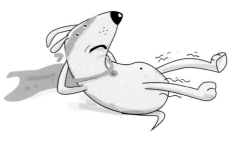

- Focus on moving slowly and mindfully, constantly asking yourself, "Could I pause here if I wanted to?"

- Check yourself and ask, "Did I fling myself here, or did I put myself here?"

- Remember that you will gain a whole lot of strength by moving between poses in a way in which you could pause and hold yourself in place at any point.

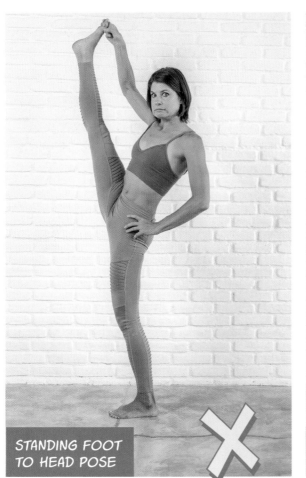

STANDING FOOT TO HEAD POSE

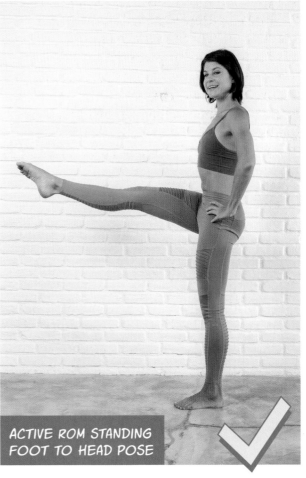

ACTIVE ROM STANDING FOOT TO HEAD POSE

Props

Maybe you're the type who goes to yoga classes and says smugly, "I don't need props." But even a yoga mat—especially a nice nonslip yoga mat—is a prop that can make certain postures easier to do passively, without activation.

There are a few common misunderstandings about when a yoga prop such as a strap or block is helping and when it's not. See if any of these scenarios sound familiar, and be cautious about any instructor's cues that encourage them:

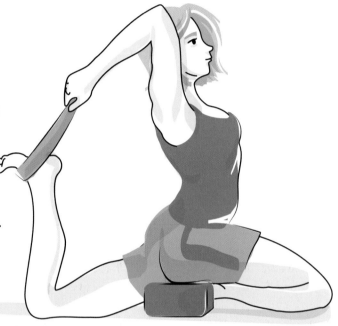

- **Using a yoga strap around your elbows in arm balances and forearm stands:** You may remember from Chapter 8 that we can benefit from strengthening our external shoulder rotators. But using a strap around our elbows makes us reliant on the strap because we're not training the external rotation that we need to eventually practice without a strap. Instead, squeeze a block or keep your feet on the floor while you work up the strength to take it into a full arm balance.

- **Using a strap to pull yourself deeper into postures:** This is the same as using your hand to pull or yank yourself deeper. Don't do it! Again, keep those muscles active.

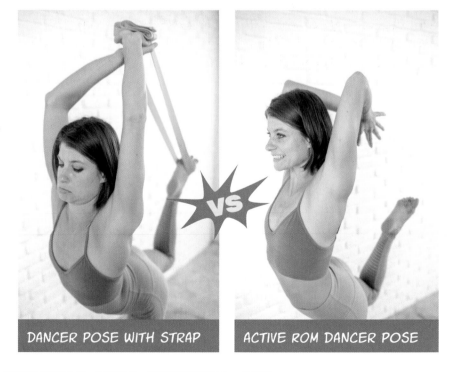

DANCER POSE WITH STRAP

ACTIVE ROM DANCER POSE

- **Relying on a block to hold you up:** Don't let the block do all the work! Make it your part-time assistant, not your full-time servant.

A good rule of thumb is that the prop is there to help make a pose more accessible, but you don't want the prop be a crutch. Always ask yourself, "Is this prop doing all the work, or am I doing the majority of the work?"

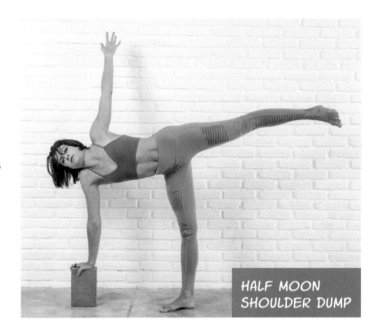

HALF MOON
SHOULDER DUMP

Off the Mat

By now, you may be thinking, "Wow, this totally changes how I practice yoga!" That's our goal, anyway—to make you more mindful of how you move. Don't stop noticing how you move when you leave your yoga class, though. Think about how you're putting yourself into positions in everyday life: Do you plop down passively onto the sofa? Can you be a bit more mindful of lowering yourself with control?

What we *don't* want you to be thinking is that you have to go through life like a robot, with all your muscles super activated all the time and never relaxed. If you're wondering, "Can I never be in my passive range of motion again? Can I ever relax?" then please, dear Bendy, read on!

Of course you can relax, and you should! It just goes back to *end range of motion.* You shouldn't ever go passively to end range of motion.

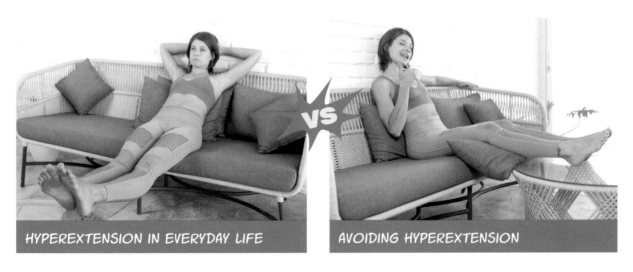

HYPEREXTENSION IN EVERYDAY LIFE

AVOIDING HYPEREXTENSION

Remember, end range is a scary place where AROM the Protector has no jurisdiction. If your muscles are relaxed and you're at end range of motion, then chances are your ligaments are stretching out and your joints will eventually experience wear and tear.[38]

JUST REMEMBER OUR NUMBER ONE SUPERPOWER TIP THAT SPANS ALL OF LIFE'S ACTIVITIES: IF YOU ARE IN PROPER POSTURE WITH YOUR S-CURVE AND PLUMB LINE INTACT, AND YOU'RE ABLE TO BREATHE NICE AND FULLY INTO YOUR LUNGS, THEN YOU'RE ALL GOOD! THIS POSTURE ISN'T POSSIBLE WITHOUT THE ACTIVATION OF THE SUPERHEROES OF THIS BOOK: THE STABILITY MUSCLES. THEY DON'T HAVE TO BE 100 PERCENT CLENCHING AND SQUEEZING TO DO THEIR JOBS; HEALTHY POSTURE ACTIVATES THEM JUST THE RIGHT AMOUNT.

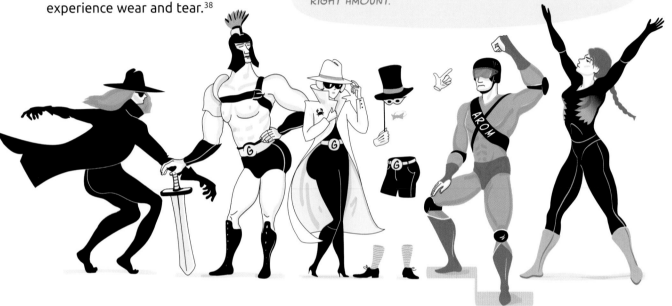

DON'T STAY IN ONE POSTURE FOR TOO LONG

"We'll stay here for three minutes. Make sure not to move."

In yin yoga classes, it's particularly important to pay attention to how you are holding your body and how gravity is pulling on your joints. Instructors' cues are often centered around being totally still for several minutes at a time and "breathing into" areas as you relax and release tension from areas of your body. While this practice can be very calming and a wonderful opportunity to relax, there's no current scientific evidence to suggest that holding a posture for longer than about 60 seconds (or just 30 seconds, according to some studies) leads to any gain in flexibility.[29]

So yin has a place, but it's not a useful way to gain flexibility, and certainly not to gain strength and stability, which we need way more of to function normally as Bendies.

While holding postures, it's important to use whatever props are necessary to ensure that your joints are *not* at end range of motion. Ask yourself, "Would there be room to move deeper if my bolster wasn't there?" If the answer is "yes," then great—you've propped yourself up enough.

We also encourage you to listen to any urges from your body to move, even if your teacher says to remain still. Evolutionarily speaking, these signals to move out of uncomfortable positions developed to protect our bodies.[192] You feel discomfort in your joints or muscles for a reason. Your body wants and needs movement.

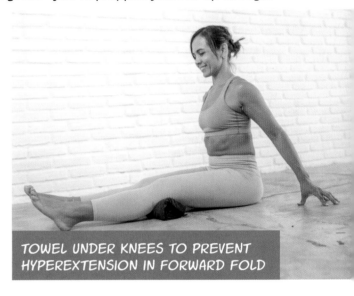

TOWEL UNDER KNEES TO PREVENT HYPEREXTENSION IN FORWARD FOLD

Even if you're in a good position when you get a signal from your body to move, it's time to move into a new position—especially because activating the stability muscles to hold yourself up can be mega tiring at first. If you catch Mr. Sloppy creeping up on you (because he is such a creep), just change positions. It's a good move to move!

Pay attention to how you feel when moving out of a posture if you've been holding it for a long time. You shouldn't experience any kind of sensation of feeling "stretched out" or feel any lethargy in your muscles. If that happens, take note that maybe you sat there for too long, and try to avoid it next time. We're always learning!

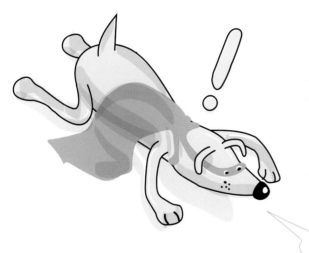

ONLY 5 MINUTES!!!

Think of an ancestor who might have been squatting under a tree to hide from the afternoon sun when a hungry tigress came along, looking for her next meal. Your ancestor wouldn't have wanted to sit in a position that would have caused their legs to go numb and wobbly, because that would have been counterproductive to the task of whisking them away to safety! We don't know about you, but we can't imagine our ancestors sitting in frog pose for 5 minutes.

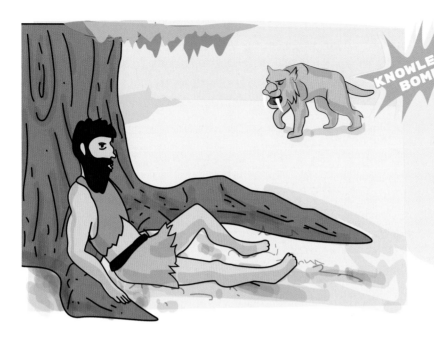

ALTHOUGH LIFE IS MUCH DIFFERENT NOW, AND THINGS THAT WERE ONCE IMPORTANT TO HUMANS AND THEIR SURVIVAL AREN'T SO IMPORTANT TO US TODAY, WE STILL HAVE THE SAME BIOLOGY. SO, LIKE IT OR NOT, WE HAVE TO RESPECT THAT BIOLOGY.

CLOSING THE GAP BETWEEN AROM AND PROM

What if there's a huge gap between where your AROM ends and your PROM ends? Well, your nervous system is in control of that, and your nervous system is like Elastidog, looking up at you with big eyes full of eagerness to learn new tricks.

You can train your nerves and tissues to be more responsive in that PROM, turning it into more range of motion that you can access *actively*.[40] KAPOW! Here's how it works.

Take, for example, a low lunge, where you reach back with an arm, grab your back foot, and pull it toward your butt. If your arm is doing all the work to pull your heel closer to your butt while your gluteus maximus is chilling with the rest of the posterior chain on the sofa binge-watching *Friends,* then that's passive. But if you leave your arm out of it entirely and just use the strength of your back leg—specifically your glutes and hamstrings—to pull your heel toward your butt, then that's active!

You can really benefit when you develop the signal to the brain that the muscles have a *purpose* in the full range of motion.

You probably can't get your foot right up to your butt without the help of your hand, so a great drill to create more neurological control in that range of motion is to put your foot in place with the help of your hand and then try to keep it there as you slowly remove your hand.

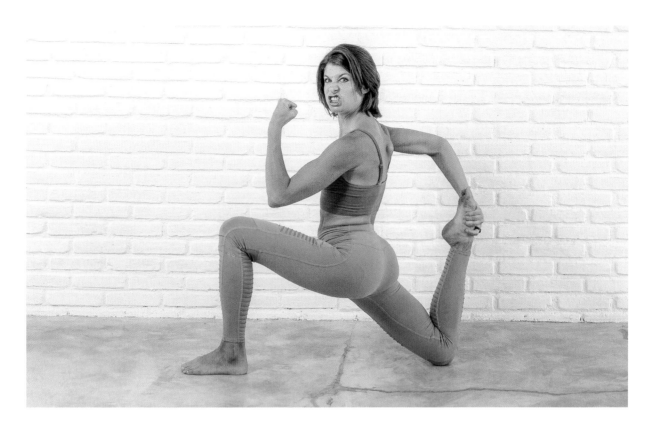

This is like sending a memo to the boss (your brain) that says, "We have discovered uncharted territory. Permission to fire in the hole." Your brain will respond, "Permission granted. Fire in the hole!" And you'll probably feel like your muscles are actually on fire (aka good pain). Yummy.

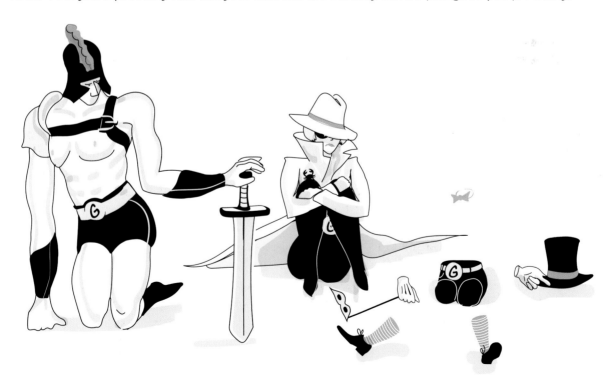

With time and practice (and by using progressive overload), your muscles will get a more robust, less-muddied-up signal to move into that range of motion without the help of your hand. It's pretty magical! Once you get super badass at that, we suggest adding a little ankle weight to take your powers to new heights.

Here's that move in detail:

- Pull your heel toward your butt as much as you can without using your hand. (*Grrr,* hello, hamstrings!)

- Then keep *allllll* those muscles that are now working hard active and switched on as you pull the foot even closer with your hand. Now you're using a combination of internal strength and external force.

- When you can't go any farther while keeping all your muscles active, try to keep your foot in place and slowly let go with your hand.

As you practice this move more and more, it'll get easier and easier. And you can do it every time you're in a yoga class and the teacher cues you to reach back and grab your foot. You can do it in so many other postures where you use an external force to deepen the posture, like the seated forward bend and camel pose mentioned earlier.

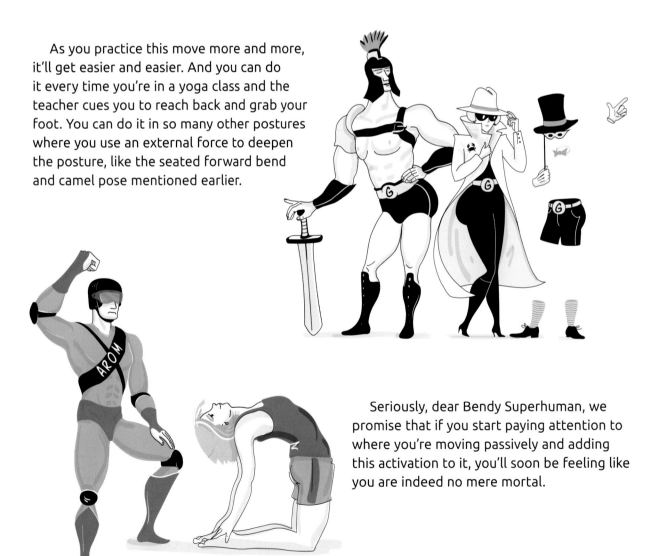

Seriously, dear Bendy Superhuman, we promise that if you start paying attention to where you're moving passively and adding this activation to it, you'll soon be feeling like you are indeed no mere mortal.

KNOWING WHEN TO MICROBEND AND WHEN NOT TO

"If you hyperextend, just put a microbend in your knees/elbows" is not a bad cue, but there's a better choice. You'll hear this cue from a lot of well-intentioned yoga teachers who recognize that hyperextending joints is not healthy. Maybe they'll even say it because they see *you,* our floppy friend, in warrior three with your standing leg losing the battle to overextension.

Putting a microbend in a joint that tends to hyperextend is definitely going to protect that joint from damage. But it's a Band-Aid. It doesn't solve the problem. The reason your joints are going into hyperextension is because *your stability muscles aren't firing.*

Knees often hyperextend because the glutes are inactive. The knees are also kept in line by other muscles, such as the tensor fasciae latae and adductor muscles. Mr. Sloppy and Sedentary Seductress are there just waiting to creep in, switch off those knee-protecting muscles, and allow your ligaments to stretch out.

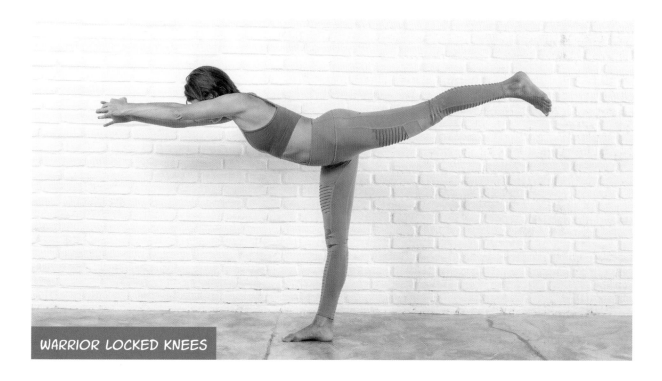

WARRIOR LOCKED KNEES

Similarly, elbows usually hyperextend because the shoulder muscles are inactive.

Training the joints to go into full extension (not hyperextension) with *muscle activation* is really good for us hypermobile people, but keep in mind that in the beginning, your muscles may fatigue at full extension. Fatigued muscles switch off. They say, "Whew, that's enough for me. I'm going to bed now. Peace out!" So move out of hyperextension into a microbend and then slowly move back toward full extension with activation, but *pay close attention* to how much you're "hanging" in that joint and how much you're actually in control. Then, if you can't hold it any longer, go back to your microbend.

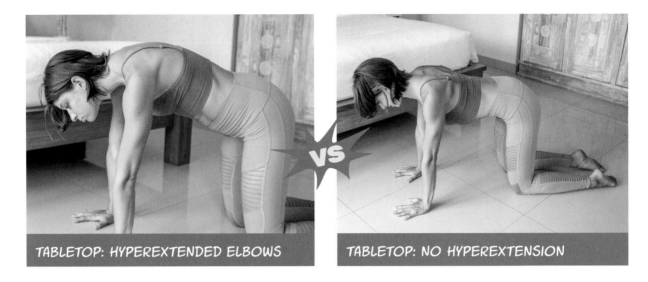

TABLETOP: HYPEREXTENDED ELBOWS   TABLETOP: NO HYPEREXTENSION

Remember progressive overload here, too. Maybe you start with just 0.1 second of muscle activation and build to longer periods of time.

REPETITIVE MOVEMENT VERSUS VARIETY

Your muscles are 3D, your body is 3D—c'mon, your whole life is 3D! So it should be obvious that moving in as many ways as possible is going to train you to be a more confident mover.

Throughout this book, we've said that we want you to keep moving and avoid sitting in any one posture for too long. The same goes for the movements between postures! A lot of yoga styles involve doing the same sequence of postures over and over again. You know by now that this approach can be great for building a skill because each time you do that sequence, you fortify the neural pathway that allows for that movement.

KNOWLEDGE BOMB!

BUT REPEATING THE SAME SEQUENCE OF POSTURES ALSO WEAKENS THE NEURAL PATHWAYS FOR OTHER MOVEMENTS.

BOOM

This is how the body and brain work. The adaptability of the nervous system is known as *neural plasticity,* and it's super cool! Interesting fact: When we took all the photos for this book and had to demonstrate all the hyperextended knees and low back hinges and bad postures, we actually found it really difficult to do! These "don'ts" were once easy and comfortable for us, but now that we've consciously trained our bodies not to hyperextend, dump, and hang in our ligaments, it feels gross and unnatural when we do.

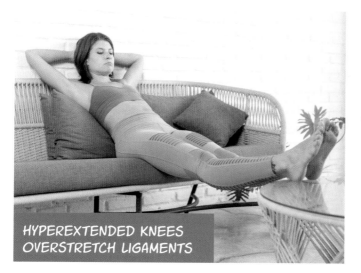

HYPEREXTENDED KNEES OVERSTRETCH LIGAMENTS

Neural plasticity can be good, bad, or neutral. But when you repeat the same sequence over and over and over again, you are reinforcing that sequence and deprioritizing other movements, taking you one step toward becoming two-dimensional. We highly encourage you to change it up a bit.

For example:

• **Chaturanga** is tough on the shoulders, and it's often done dozens of times in a single yoga practice. Ouch! So change it up each time you do it. Externally rotate your hands, move your arms out wider than your shoulders, or lower your knees. You can practice chaturanga by going just one-tenth of the way down, or three-quarters of the way, or go beyond that beloved 90-degree elbow angle that yoga teachers always cue.

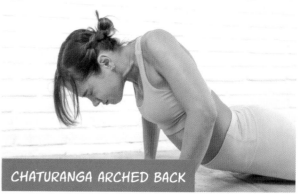

CHATURANGA ARCHED BACK

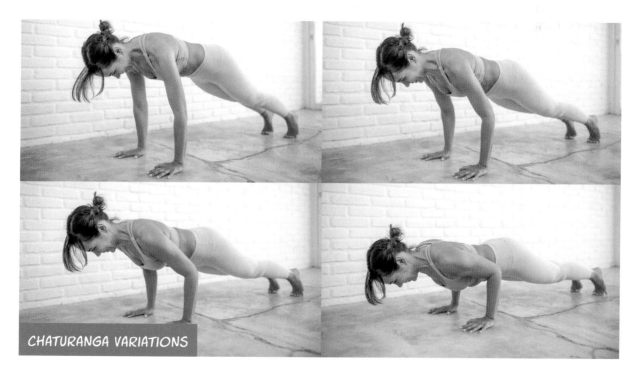

CHATURANGA VARIATIONS

- **Sun salutations** can be varied in a million ways to give your body new options. Here are three ideas: take your feet wide to the edges of your mat, do it on one leg, or start at the end and go backward. Can you think of any of the remaining 999,997 variations?

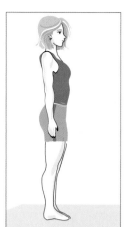
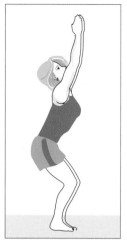
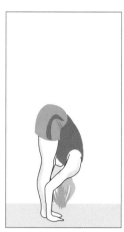

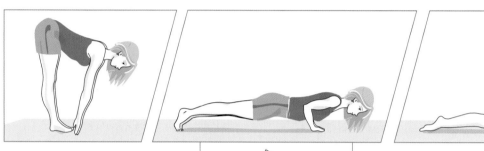

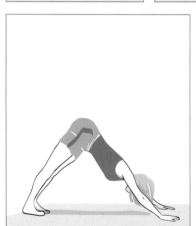
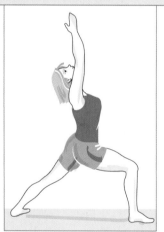
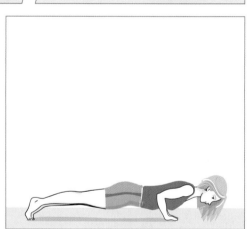

As biomechanist and author Katy Bowman says, movement is nutrition, just like food. So make sure to get a varied movement diet!

Varying your movements involves not just the range of motion and the directions and shapes you go into and out of, but also how quickly or slowly you move and the amount of load you move with.

We like to think of all the ways in which a ninja would move: running, jumping, kicking, swinging, and twirling, but also stealthily moving through the shadows, slowly creeping, and holding totally still to avoid being noticed. That ninja can perform such a wide variety of movements because there are fibers and cells and electrical charges in the body to allow for those different types of movement. All humans have the ability to move in many ways because movement is built into us! But if we don't train it, those tissues and cells can atrophy, forget why they're there, and become weak.

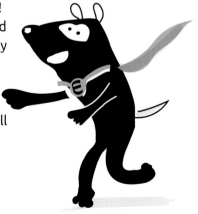

As yogis, we spend a lot of time practicing slow movements and static postures, but we rarely call upon our more explosive, fast-moving muscle fibers. If you're into other types of exercise that involve running, jumping, or kicking, then you're probably pretty well rounded in this department. However, a lot of yoga addicts don't do anything but yoga, and if you belong to this group, then adding explosive movements like bouncing and jumping to your practice will accelerate your superhuman training.

These kinds of movements work a property of our soft tissues (muscles, tendons, and other soft tissues) called *elasticity*.

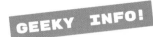

ELASTICITY

THE HUMAN BODY IS ABLE TO RUN, JUMP, BOUNCE, QUICKLY CHANGE DIRECTIONS, AND LEAP THANKS TO THE ELASTICITY OF OUR TISSUES.

ELASTICITY ISN'T REALLY ABOUT FLEXIBILITY OR STRENGTH. IT'S MORE ABOUT THE ABILITY TO RECOIL TO A SHAPE AFTER BEING DEFORMED (STRETCHED). THIS TRAIT ALLOWS FOR RESILIENCE AND LONGEVITY. ONE THING THAT ALLOWS FOR GREATER ELASTICITY IS TENSION--SOMETHING HYPERMOBILE PEOPLE OFTEN LACK.

IMAGINE AN 8-INCH PIECE OF RUBBER BAND AND AN 8-INCH PIECE OF BUNGEE CORD. THE RUBBER BAND IS MUCH MORE FLEXIBLE AND FLOPPY. HOLDING THE RUBBER BAND IN BOTH HANDS AND STRETCHING IT DOESN'T REQUIRE MUCH EFFORT AT ALL. STRETCHING THE BUNGEE CORD, HOWEVER, TAKES A LOT MORE EFFORT, RIGHT? BECAUSE IT'S MUCH TIGHTER!

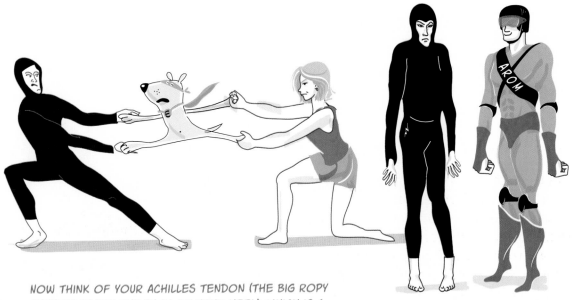

NOW THINK OF YOUR ACHILLES TENDON (THE BIG ROPY TENDON ABOVE THE BACK OF YOUR HEEL), WHICH IS A MAJOR PLAYER IN RUNNING AND JUMPING. IF YOUR ACHILLES WERE LIKE A RUBBER BAND, WOULD YOU BE ABLE TO JUMP AS HIGH OR RUN AS EASILY? NO. YOU WANT YOUR ACHILLES TENDON TO BE MORE LIKE A BUNGEE CORD.

SO BASICALLY, THE MORE TENSION A TENDON HAS, THE GREATER ITS ABILITY TO BOUNCE.

Hypermobile people often struggle to bounce or jump high, and they run with greater effort than a lot of their stiffer hypomobile friends because hypermobility often causes a laxity in the tissues that help us bounce. If the tendons don't have this recoil ability due to tension, then muscles have to do more work. And that's tiring!

But nothing is forever; we are not stuck with bodies that don't want to recoil quickly. Like anything, we can train our ability to jump and bounce.[230]

We want to drill into your head that above all else, it's important to move in a way that tells your brain everything is "safe." So if you're working to build new habits and break old ones in the posture department, or perhaps you're making an effort to replace Mr. Sloppy with AROM the Protector and move with greater stability through your joints, then move as slowly as you need to while you learn that new way of moving.

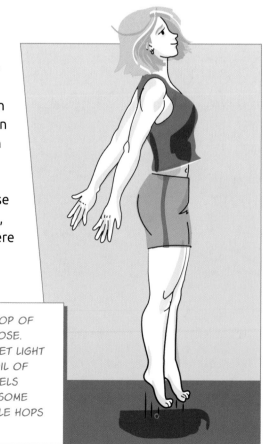

To get your brain fully on board, remember that you need to add intensity through progressive overload. We recommend keeping your movements slow at first but adding some weight. However, once your body and brain are like, "Ohhh...got it. We're doing it like this now," then adding speed is a great way to develop greater strength and coordination.

Consider some of the slow movements you make in your yoga practice and think of some ways to make those movements a bit quicker to challenge your coordination, your balance, and your superhuman muscle strength. Here are some examples we love:

> ADD A LITTLE BOUNCING SESSION AT THE TOP OF YOUR SUN SALUTATION IN YOUR STANDING POSE. SHIFT YOUR WEIGHT TO YOUR TOES AND GET LIGHT ON YOUR HEELS. USING THE NATURAL RECOIL OF YOUR ACHILLES TENDON, BOUNCE YOUR HEELS UP AND DOWN. IF THIS FEELS GOOD, GET SOME AIRTIME AND TURN THE BOUNCES INTO LITTLE HOPS OR EVEN BIG JUMPS.

FROM YOUR CRESCENT LUNGE, STEP YOUR BACK FOOT FORWARD, BRINGING YOUR KNEE TO YOUR CHEST, AND THEN STEP BACK TO YOUR LUNGE. MAKE THE MOVEMENT OF BRINGING YOUR KNEE TO YOUR CHEST FASTER AS YOU GAIN CONFIDENCE IN IT, AS IF YOU'RE USING YOUR KNEE TO KARATE-CHOP ALL THE VILLAINS IN THIS BOOK! IF YOU'RE FEELING GOOD THERE, ADD A LITTLE BOUNCE, HOP, OR JUMP OFF OF YOUR BOTTOM FOOT AS YOU BRING YOUR KNEE UP.

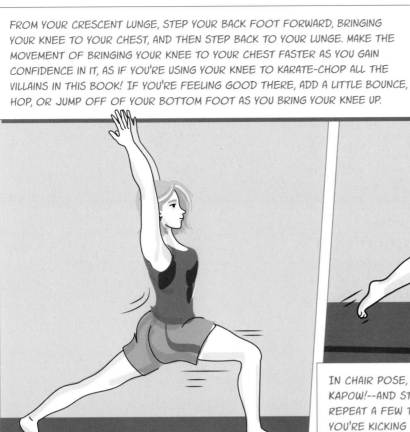

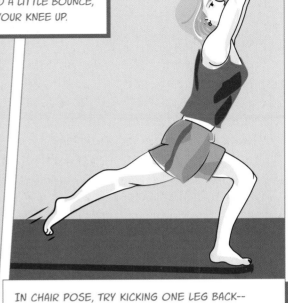

IN CHAIR POSE, TRY KICKING ONE LEG BACK-- KAPOW!--AND STEPPING IT BACK TO CHAIR POSE. REPEAT A FEW TIMES WITH BOTH LEGS AS IF YOU'RE KICKING AWAY ALL THE ANNOYING THINGS IN YOUR LIFE THAT YOU DON'T WANT ANYMORE.

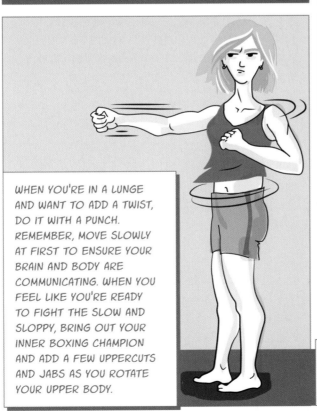

WHEN YOU'RE IN A LUNGE AND WANT TO ADD A TWIST, DO IT WITH A PUNCH. REMEMBER, MOVE SLOWLY AT FIRST TO ENSURE YOUR BRAIN AND BODY ARE COMMUNICATING. WHEN YOU FEEL LIKE YOU'RE READY TO FIGHT THE SLOW AND SLOPPY, BRING OUT YOUR INNER BOXING CHAMPION AND ADD A FEW UPPERCUTS AND JABS AS YOU ROTATE YOUR UPPER BODY.

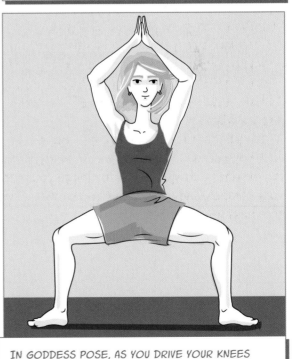

IN GODDESS POSE, AS YOU DRIVE YOUR KNEES BACK, ADD SOME BOUNCES. WANT TO FEEL LIKE A REAL BADASS? TURN YOUR BOUNCES TO JUMPS.

SAY GOODBYE TO SOME OTHER BAD CUES

Finally, we'd like to revisit two bad cues. These cues have already been mentioned in previous chapters, but it's worth looking at them again here because of their prevalence in the yoga world.

"Draw your shoulders down and back..."

This is a great cue for upward-facing dog or chin-ups, but if your arms are raised overhead, then *you must ignore this cue.*

When your arms are raised overhead, such as in

- Chair pose
- Lunging postures
- Tree pose

or when your arms are overhead and bearing weight in inverted postures, such as

- Dolphin pose
- Downward-facing dog
- Handstand

the natural movement of the shoulder joint means that your shoulders will rise toward your ears! Think about reaching up to change a light bulb or retrieve a plate from a high shelf. You wouldn't try to keep your shoulder down away from your ear.

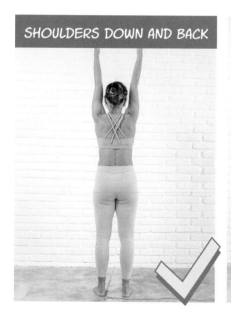

SHOULDERS DOWN AND BACK

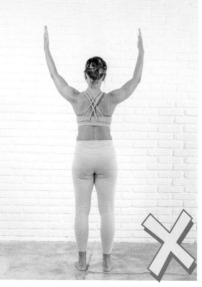

Furthermore, when bearing weight as in downward-facing dog, you are using your *pushing* muscles. When you pull your shoulders away from your ears, you are...well, pulling! Save that motion for your pull-ups.

Still not sure? Go back and review the information on shoulder stability in Chapter 7.

"Relax your glutes"

We discussed this already, but no matter how many times we tell people, "Keep your glutes active in backbends," they still ask us, "But what about *[insert every backbending posture]*?" And we wonder how many more times we will need to say it to make it sink in.

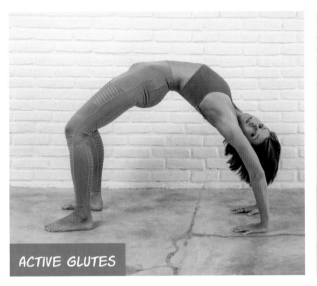
ACTIVE GLUTES

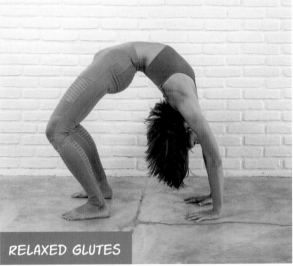
RELAXED GLUTES

Honestly, we don't know of any time when it would be good to purposefully relax your glutes except when you're in your savasana or you're on a massage table getting an elbow to your butt cheeks from your favorite massage therapist.

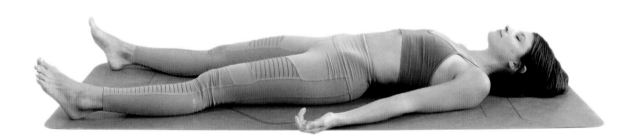

The glutes are the biggest muscles in the body, and their role is to stabilize the pelvis. The pelvis—don't forget—is right there in the middle of your body, so the position of your pelvis *will* affect your low back and knees as well as implicate the alignment of your shoulders, your feet, and even your jaw![162,193]

So, when you go into *any* backbend, what you are doing is *extending your hips*. That means you are moving your legs posteriorly (behind your hips). This action is done through the glutes—or at least it should be. If you relax your glutes in a backbend, you risk harming your lower back.

"But when I squeeze my glutes in a backbend, it actually hurts my back more."

If this statement sounds familiar, check whether you're properly activating your glutes. What often happens when the glutes become weak is that they simply don't fire, even when we tell them to. We think, "*Squeeeeze* that peach!" and, due to years of improper glute activation, what we are actually doing is getting our low back muscles to do the work of the glutes.[125]

Have a feel of your butt to see if you can get the actual booty muscles to activate. Use that activation to keep your pelvis stable in your backbends and lunges.[143]

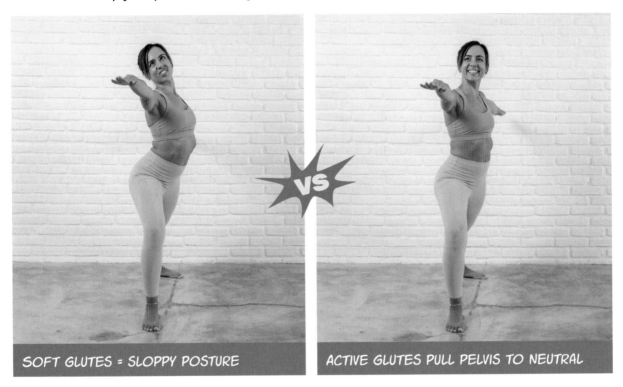

SOFT GLUTES = SLOPPY POSTURE

ACTIVE GLUTES PULL PELVIS TO NEUTRAL

"So am I supposed to walk around like a robot with my butt clenched all the time?"

No! Think about this: do your quads and calves activate when you're walking? Sure as hell they do! Otherwise, you wouldn't be upright. But you don't consciously squeeze or clench your quads or calves when you're walking unless you're trying to do the robot. They are able to activate to the amount that's needed to allow you to take each step. If you're walking uphill, your quads will work a bit harder without you even thinking about it.

Ideally, the glutes do the same. If your glutes are like lazy couch potatoes that want to slouch around all day, however, you may have to consciously wake them up at first. One great place to start is with your backbends.

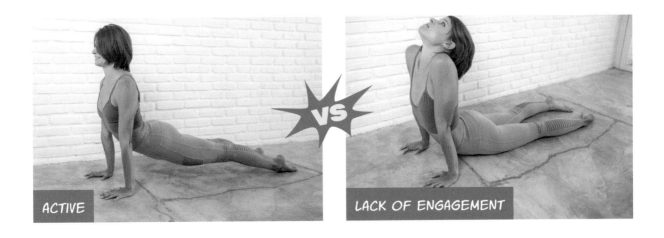

ACTIVE   VS   LACK OF ENGAGEMENT

LOVE FOR THE YOGA TEACHERS AND FITNESS INSTRUCTORS WHO ARE JUST DOING THEIR BEST

As long as you stay hungry and curious, you're a hero.

You probably know by now that what we want any hypermobile person to be thinking about, focusing on, and working on is building strength around their joints. Strength comes through time, patience, and practice. And *yes,* your yoga practice *can* be a great way to build strength.

Let's leave the injuries to the extreme sports fanatics and freak accidents from now on, shall we?

Yoga teachers are doing *great work*. And teaching yoga is so hard. You yoga teachers out there are nodding your heads in agreement, are we right?

The effort to put a class together; remember your sequence; cue that sequence to a room full of people with different bodies and abilities; command the attention of all those people; be mindful of your playlist, the time, and the temperature of the room; and give hands-on assists to your students—all while doing your best to give everyone an enjoyable experience—is *significant*.

We yoga teachers sometimes make mistakes. We say the wrong thing, and we give cues that aren't helpful to everyone.

But above all, yoga is an *inward journey to understand yourself,* and that's why being able to hear certain cues and know how to modify for your body's needs is very much a part of the practice!

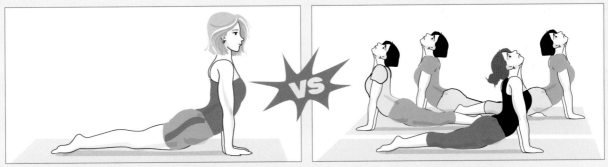

As Adell always tells her students, "Listen to your body, and let your body's voice be louder than mine." Yoga teachers are merely guides. Your true guru is your body.

CHAPTER 11:

ANXIOUS ABOUT HYPERMOBILITY?

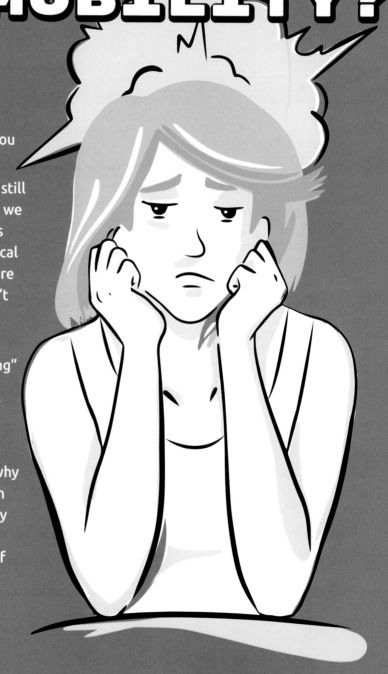

Your hypermobility may be making you anxious.

The thing is, there's just so much we still don't know about the body. By "we," we mean humans in general, the authors of this book included. Even top medical experts and renowned biochemists are unable to answer questions that don't seem all that complex.

If you're in the "this-is-the-twenty-first-century-and-we-know-everything" camp, we dare you to go find a definitive answer for why the skin of our fingers wrinkles in water or why we have fingerprints. There are only theories for why men have nipples, why we sometimes have random itches on our skin from no known cause, or why the right brain controls the left side of the body and vice versa. The list of "unknowns" goes on and on!

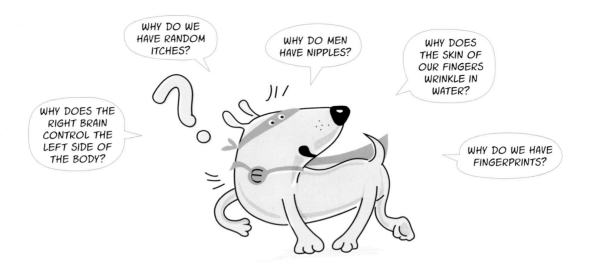

Delve into the world of biology for just a few minutes, and all you'll find is evidence of our ignorance and how good we are at merely speculating.

So we think it's worth taking a moment to be in awe of your body—even if it does cause you pain and anxiety—for how beautifully complex it is. Respect the delicately balanced entanglement of cells, hormones, bacteria, and all the other stuff—known and unknown—that make up this vessel. Revere how, after eons of having these bodies, we still can't understand them, let alone manufacture any machine that comes even reasonably close to replicating what our bodies do each and every day.

So how *does* hypermobility lead to anxiety?

> FILE THAT ONE UNDER "WE'RE NOT SURE." WE JUST CALL IT THE PANIC MECHANIC, ANOTHER DREADED VILLAIN THAT WE BENDIES HAVE TO BATTLE.

But there are people who have devoted themselves to finding the answer. Several studies show that anxiety is more prevalent among the hypermobile population, and we know that this type of anxiety is physiological—meaning it's not in your head but in your body.[7]

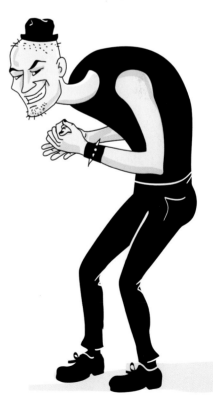

POSSIBLE CAUSES OF ANXIETY IN BENDY PEOPLE

One explanation for why hypermobility comes with a higher causality to anxiety is that the stretchiness of the blood vessels creates a pooling of blood—that is, the walls of the vessels lack the tension to withstand the pressure of the blood rushing through, so the blood isn't pushed through as quickly as it should be. Remember, hypermobility doesn't just make you extra stretchy in your muscles, tendons, and ligaments; it affects all of your soft tissues, including your blood vessels.

So imagine that, instead of being in a normal toothpaste tube, your toothpaste is housed in a balloon. As you try to push the toothpaste out of the balloon to smear it onto your toothbrush, the stretchiness of the balloon allows the toothpaste to spread out, pressing the sides of the balloon outward instead of being forced in one direction.

The effect in blood vessels that lack the normal tautness is similar.

So, when our blood begins to pool, our bodies react with—**dun-dun-dun-DUUUN**—adrenaline! This chemical, normally reserved for high-intensity situations—like…oh, *almost dying*—is how our bodies help blood move more quickly through our stretchy veins and arteries.[194] The result is that we feel like we're having a near-death experience for no reason.[19] So totally boring not-deathly experiences like walking to work and ordering food at a restaurant make us feel all quivery and jittery.

Is it at all surprising that this nonstop IV drip of adrenaline is basically an enormous welcome mat for the Panic Mechanic?

If you're feeling mind-blown right now, just wait; it gets even more interesting. Another explanation for the higher prevalence of anxiety among the hypermobile population is that hypermobility leads to increased sensitivity.[7] *This is another superpower in disguise!*

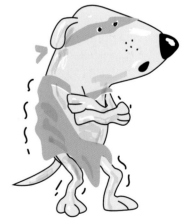

Some research shows that hypermobile people have heightened awareness of their external environment as well as what's happening within their bodies.[231] This includes nociception, which is the proper word for the perception of threat, and that leads to the sensation of pain.[7] So, if you've ever been told that you're "too sensitive" or called a "highly sensitive person," you may be saying "ooooooh" right about now. Again, it's not in your head. It's in your body—in your stretchy tissues, to be (kind of) exact.

> Pain, and the perception of pain, is a very interesting subject to dig into if you're interested. You can download a free PDF of *Recovery Strategies: Your Pain Guidebook* at www.greglehman.ca/pain-science-workbooks.

There are also cases of superhumans-in-training being treated for cervical spine instability that compresses the vagus nerve. Basically, the lack of stability in the neck means that the bones of the spine there push on one of the most important nerves in the body.[19] The vagus nerve is like the momma nerve for the parasympathetic nervous system—the part of the nervous system that allows us to rest, digest, and repair.[195] Stimulation of the vagus nerve therefore leads to feelings of calm, but if a person's vagus nerve isn't able to transmit those calming messages to the rest of the body, then it's easy to see how that person might remain in an anxious, stressed-out state.

We think it's wise to assume that any anxiety you feel is the result of some unknown combination of these factors plus others, such as your external environment and any stressful situations you may be dealing with.

Maybe one day we humans will be able to pinpoint the specific origins of anxiety in each individual, but at the time of writing this book, it's still quite the head-scratcher. So the link between anxiety and hypermobility is understandably extra head-scratcher-y.

But in a way, it doesn't really matter why the anxiety is there; what's more important is to understand *what to do about it.*

While we certainly want to minimize the suffering caused by anxiety, remember that suffering and sensation are two different things. You can feel anxious, and you can be aware of the effects of anxiety on your body, mind, and mood, but you do not have to suffer. Of course, it's not easy, and it takes work—daily work. And perhaps the hardest thing is the fact that the world we live in isn't built for managing anxiety. Our world and the lifestyles we are encouraged to live are in most ways incongruent with the needs of a person living with anxiety. It's often difficult to feel understood or heard, so it's no fun. But through all that, you still do not have to suffer.

You have within you, every second of your life, an amazing and powerful tool: your breath.

Sometimes we think of the human body as a complex machine made up of a mishmash of individual parts and gears all working simultaneously, and in some ways, that's a good way to think about it. But we prefer to think of each cell in the body (human and otherwise*) as being like an individual person working for a really big logistics company. Within that company are various teams that specialize in different areas of the business, with bosses, bosses' bosses, and bosses' bosses' bosses. And the nervous system is like the company's email network. From the intern who just got hired to do the filing and restock the printer ink cartridges to the CEO who's making all the key decisions, everyone in the company has an email address and is able to send and receive messages. This helps ensure that important messages are communicated to the right people.

When you count all the bacteria that make up the microbiome that keeps your body functions running, the majority of cells in your body are actually nonhuman.

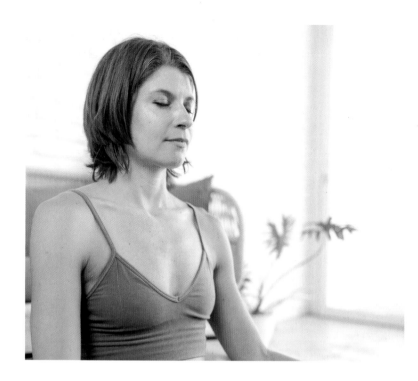

Anxiety is like a rumor going around that the company's finances are in trouble and the board is going to let a bunch of the staff go—a rumor that's false.

Your breath is the way to send an email to all the employees of the company that says, "Relax! Everything's good, and all your jobs are safe! In fact, you're all getting a pay raise!" That's because your breath is the easiest way to stimulate the vagus nerve, and thus the parasympathetic nervous system, your calm and restful state.[197]

BREATHING TO EASE ANXIETY

For your next ten breaths, open your mouth and take very short, shallow, and quick sips of air while bracing the muscles of your belly so tightly that you can breathe only into the top portion of your lungs.

How do you feel?

Now, through your nose, inhale slowly over a count of six, allowing your lungs to fill downward toward your belly, out to the sides of your rib cage, to the front and back of your ribs, and upward. Now exhale slowly through your nose over another count of six.

Feel a difference?

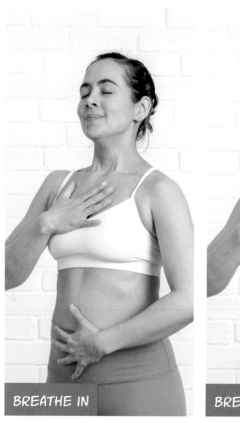

BREATHE IN

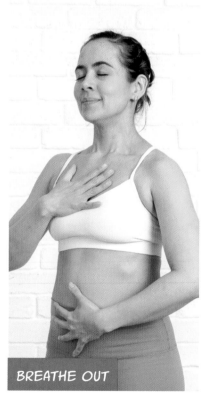

BREATHE OUT

The breath is powerful! We overlook its power because it's always there, even while we sleep. And, let's face it, no Olympic medals are awarded for great breathing, nor are magazine covers selling us images of lungs that are optimally utilized.

But imagine we live in a world where millions of adoring fans follow great breathers on Instagram, and you might overhear someone say in the gym, "Hey, man, your breathing is impressive!" We imagine that people would be much happier and healthier in this world. In our actual world, most people aren't breathing optimally.

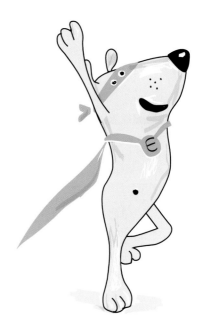

Just as you may have experienced in the mini breathing activity we suggested, how you breathe controls how you *feel*.

The 360-degree nasal breath that we just described is encouraged in yoga classes, where some of us may, for the first time in our lives, unknowingly learn the skill of breathing properly. Even when things get challenging, we yogis know to keep breathing through the nose. A classic sign of a first-time yoga practitioner is huffing and puffing with O-shaped lips when the vinyasas get intense.

Our mouths really aren't meant for breathing. When we breathe through our noses, several things happen:

- The nostrils and nasal cavities filter, moisten, and warm the air we inhale before it enters the lungs.[205]

- The smaller and more meandering nasal passageways force us to breathe more slowly, which prevents the loss of carbon dioxide (CO_2). CO_2 is responsible for oxygen being released into our cells. Even though our cells live on oxygen, they need CO_2 to help the blood deliver that oxygen! If we breathe too quickly, we exhale the CO_2 that our cells need.[206]

- An enzyme in our sinuses produces nitric oxide, which is delivered to the lungs and carried into the bloodstream. Nitric oxide is hugely important for optimal cell function because it allows for the dilation of the blood vessels (known as vasodilation).[207]

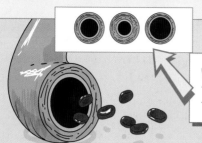

VASODILATION = BETTER BLOOD FLOW TO THE ORGANS = BETTER FUNCTION OF THE ORGANS AND MUSCLES

BETTER BRAIN FUNCTION = IMPROVED MEMORY AND FOCUS, LIKE REMEMBERING THAT EVERYTHING IS FINE AND FOCUSING ON HOW MANY THINGS IN LIFE ARE GREAT = DECREASED ANXIETY

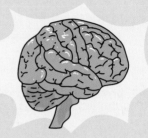

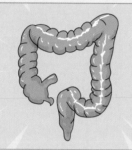

BETTER GUT FUNCTION = BETTER ABSORPTION OF NUTRIENTS AND REGULATION OF HORMONES = BETTER OVERALL BALANCE OF YOUR BODY

BETTER MUSCLE FUNCTION = IMPROVED PERFORMANCE IN WHATEVER YOU'RE DOING = LESS PAIN AND INJURY

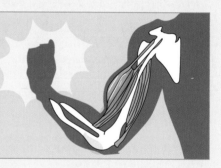

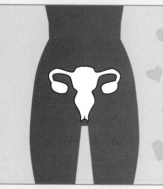

BETTER SEX ORGAN FUNCTION = BETTER ERECTIONS AND ORGASMS = EVERYONE'S HAPPY

BETTER IMMUNE FUNCTION = BETTER DEFENSE AGAINST HARMFUL INVADERS = BETTER HEALTH

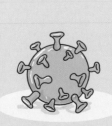

We hope that at this point, you're breathing through your nose and allowing your belly to expand with each inhalation! Can you carry this type of breathing into every aspect of your life?

Even when your heart rate is elevated because you're frustrated with your doctor for not taking you seriously when you say you think your anxiety is linked to your hypermobility, we encourage you to breathe through your nose as much as possible. Like anything, it gets easier with practice.

For now, just pay attention to how you're breathing, especially when you start to feel the Panic Mechanic working away at you. If you're in a stressful situation or feeling frustrated, get into the habit of focusing on your breath and bringing it to those long, slow, expansive inhales and exhales through your nose.

ADDITIONAL RESOURCES ABOUT BREATHING

All sorts of cool chemical stuff happens in our bodies when we breathe in different ways. As much as we would love to go into that, we want to keep this book simple. You can check out the following resources if you want to get geeky about the breath and exactly *how* it all happens:

The Oxygen Advantage: The Simple, Scientifically Proven Breathing Techniques for a Healthier, Slimmer, Faster, and Fitter You

by Patrick McKeown

Activate Your Vagus Nerve: Unleash Your Body's Natural Ability to Heal

by Dr. Navaz Habib

Exhale: 40 Breathwork Exercises to Help You Find Your Calm, Supercharge Your Health, and Perform at Your Best

by Richie Bostock

ANXIETY AND NEURAL PLASTICITY

So let's recap. Bendy People are more prone to anxiety because

- Our stretchy blood vessels lead to overkill on the adrenaline.[198]

- We're more sensitive to pain and those inexplicable "gut feelings."[8,68]

- Our floppy posture may be inhibiting some nerves from signaling properly.

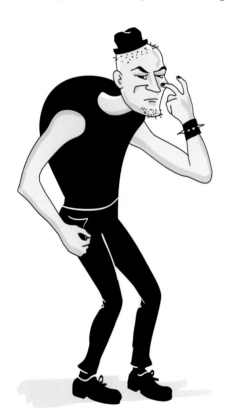

As far as we know, there's no way to make your blood vessels or ligaments more taut. But that hardly matters when you understand the power of—**ANGELS SINGING**—*neural plasticity,* which is basically what we've been talking about throughout this book: changing habits and patterns.[36]

KNOWLEDGE BOMB!

IT'S OUR PATTERNS THAT ARE LETTING US DOWN, NOT OUR BODIES. AND OUR HABITS ARE WHAT FORM OUR PATTERNS.

BOOM!

It all starts in the nervous system, remember? Every move you make, every breath you take, creepy Mr. Sloppy is watching you. (Just kidding.) Every function of the body occurs because the nervous system has neurological patterns in place for that function, and the nervous system is constantly adapting and changing. You are not stuck with anything.

You're not stuck with floppy joints. You're not stuck with anxious thoughts. You're not stuck with posture that leaves you achy. And you're certainly not stuck in any situation that you want to change.

It's time to introduce Guru Gumshoe, the detective living within us all, to discover our unique needs and quirks. Ultimately, science isn't yet advanced enough to answer all the questions we have as individuals. The body and mind and how everything works together are just *tooooo* complex for Google, doctors, or this book to answer all your questions. So let your inner Guru

Gumshoe get to work to decipher the things that trigger you, the things that calm you, the circumstances that help you, and the experiences that hinder your ability to fight off the Panic Mechanic. We believe that the only real guru is you, and you're only a guru to yourself. So get to work, Guru Gumshoe; start to see everything related to your anxiety as a mystery to be solved, a coded message to be decrypted.

To allow your Guru Gumshoe to do its job effectively, you need to follow some simple steps.

Step 1: Stop listening to your mind

Your mind is ruled by your ego and by the information overload that surrounds you everywhere you go. In other words, your mind is like a bratty teenager who thinks she knows everything about how the world works because she watched a couple of YouTube videos.

Your body, though, is NATURE. Humankind has been evolving for, like, a gazillion years, and with all that time comes a wisdom in your body that your mind simply can't comprehend. Humans, with our space travel and have-whatever-we-can-dream-of-delivered-to-our-doors technology, are actually still baffled by a lot of the workings of the body. Meanwhile, your body's like, "You'll understand when you're older, kiddo."

So, to heed the wise words of your body, just stop listening to your bratty teenager mind.

Pay attention to when your decisions are based on what you're *thinking* rather than how you're *feeling*. For example, are you doing a deep backbend in yoga class because your ego is telling you it'll look really cool, whereas your lower back is like, "Umm, can we not?" Or perhaps you find yourself grabbing a snack because your brain says it's time to eat and not because you feel hungry.

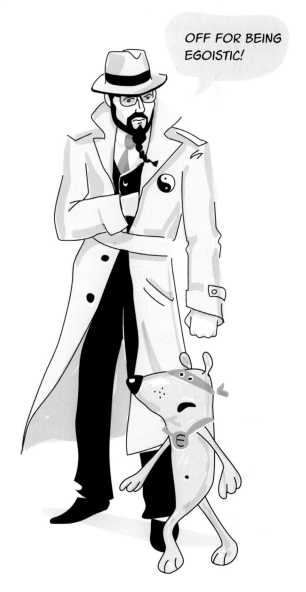

Step 2: Experiment

That wordless language of the human body means it's sometimes hard to decipher what the body is asking for. It speaks to us with pain, energy, fatigue, great moods, crappy moods, brain-fog, alertness, bloating, good sleep, bad sleep—you get the picture.

To figure out what your body is telling you, you have to try different things and pay attention—with a mindset of a scientist in a research lab—to which foods, movements, or other experiences repeatedly lead you to feel great. Experimenting and observing the results is the number one way to start heeding your guru's advice.

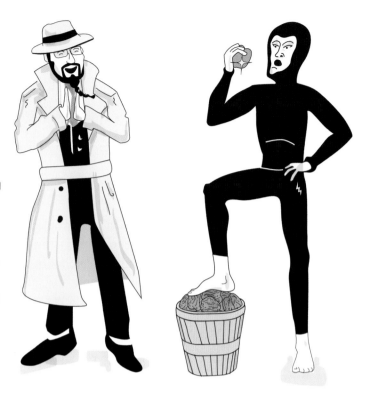

Step 3: Be Present

We're usually in a rush to have our questions answered, our problems remedied, and our dreams turned into reality. But remember that although our minds are swept up in the current of the fast-paced technology-driven world around us, our bodies are on a different current—the slower flowing rhythm of nature.

One trap you may regularly fall into is to want your body to do *all the things NOW*. To be healed from injury NOW. To detoxify from that indulgent weekend NOW. And because it doesn't happen STRAIGHTAWAY, your mind may get all control-freakish and come up with ways to expedite these things.

In reality, if you simply have some patience and pay attention to how you're feeling NOW, then you're better able to listen to exactly what is going on with your body.

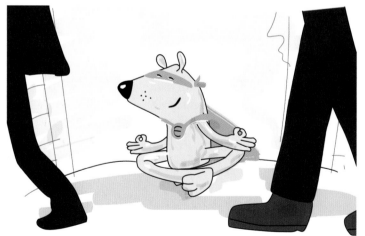

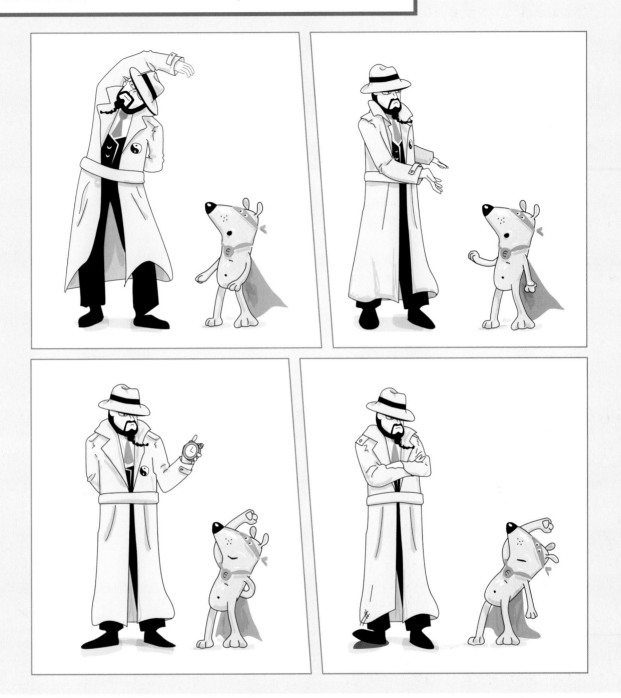

Like anything, these steps take practice, and it is very much a journey of continuous learning! Your body is constantly adapting, and that means its language is always changing slightly. But that's what makes it so profoundly beautiful!

For more on this subject, we highly recommend the book *The Brain That Changes Itself: Stories of Personal Triumph from the Frontiers of Brain Science* by Norman Doidge, which tells dozens of stories of people changing their situations through neural plasticity.

CHAPTER 12:

HYPERMOBILITY AND GUT ISSUES

NOTE: MOST OF THIS BOOK IS FROM A SHARED PERSPECTIVE, WITH BOTH OF US CONTRIBUTING. MUCH OF THIS CHAPTER, HOWEVER, IS WRITTEN FROM ADELL'S PERSPECTIVE AND REFLECTS HER EXPERIENCE.

I am kind of obsessed with digestion. It's easy to obsess about something that doesn't function properly in your body.

But then, what is proper gut functioning? To understand that, we can ask these questions: What is the purpose of the digestive system, and what should it be doing for us?

In a nutshell, the answer to that question is *to break down our food into nutrients for our cells to do their manifold jobs, and to get rid of waste that's of no use to our cells.*

In truth, it's way more complex than that, but those are the fundamentals. The more efficiently your food gets turned into useful nutrients and energy, the better your gut is functioning. So "gut issues" can include anything that disrupts that function.

My gut was not functioning optimally. I began to wonder, "Why is my poop always runny, and why do I get painful bloating after eating certain foods? And is it okay that I sometimes see undigested bits of food in my poop?" Naturally, I thought, "I'll go to a doctor and find out!" Over the next several years, I saw doctors in the US, the UK, and Australia. I had blood tests and stool tests. Every doctor gave me the same dismissive response, something akin to "Why are you here? You're not unwell."

In our experience, going to a doctor with a long list of annoying but not life-threatening symptoms results in, at best, a polite "If anything gets worse, come back and see me."

For sure, one of the villains not just of hypermobility but of Western medicine in general is the failure to recognize the interconnectedness of everything and the pure *brilliance* of the human body's ability to regulate itself. Those annoying-but-not-life-threatening issues are the body's way of meekly saying, "Ahem, sorry to bother you, but...could we perhaps try something different? This isn't working for me."

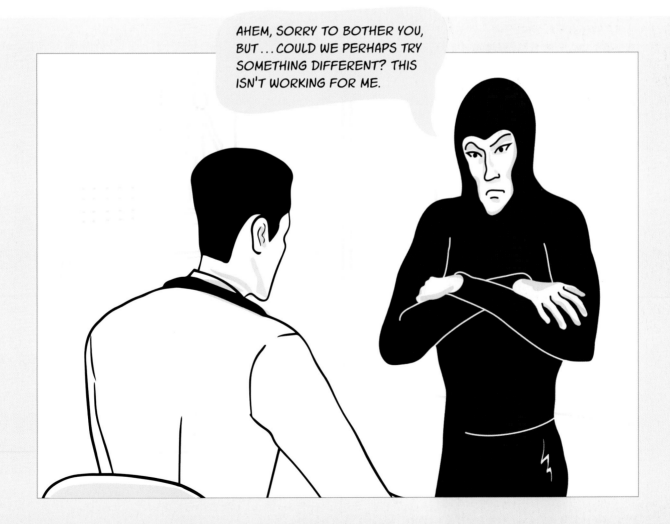

Your body will carry on with those annoying issues for months or years, or maybe even decades, until it decides that enough is enough and starts screaming, "I can't take it anymore!" The result is much more extreme issues.

Maybe you're there already. Maybe you just have some slight annoyances. I, you must know, am a bit of a princess and don't like to feel even the slightest discomfort. So it didn't take me long to proclaim, "I don't like this. I want to feel *amazing* all the time."

Thus began my obsession with my digestion and my quest to figure out the problem myself.

You may remember Guru Gumshoe from Chapter 11. I realized that this super detective is good at investigating more than just anxiety; I employed Guru Gumshoe for my gut issues, too.

My issues weren't limited to runny poop and bloating. I had feelings of lethargy and weakness despite eating a healthy and balanced diet and sleeping loads. I had cystic acne all over my face. I felt uncertain about every meal because I didn't know what would be okay and what might cause hours of painful bloating. Thankfully, those days are now in the past for me.

One thing I learned as I delved into the wonders of digestion is that the body's ability to digest food efficiently can and will affect every single thing about the body, from hormones to hair loss and from mood to memory.

BENDY PERSON BELLY PROBLEMS

It's not unusual for Bendy People to have very different experiences than their non-bendy friends, such as indigestion or acid reflux, not to mention differences in how things come out the other end. Digestive issues that correlate higher with hypermobility make up a long list:[208]

- Abdominal wall tears

- Acid reflux

- Bloating

- Constipation

- Delayed gastric emptying

- Diarrhea

- Hiatal hernia

- Leaky gut

- Painful gas

- And almost any other issue related to the digestive system

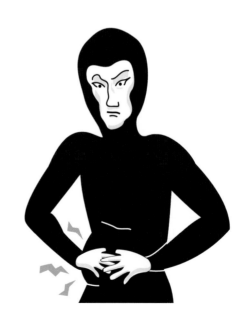

To avoid getting into the science-y nitty-gritty that we know you ain't got time for, we'll keep it simple: you may be experiencing digestive issues because, like so many other things in your body, **your digestive organs are too stretchy.**[208]

Think about it: if your esophagus is too stretchy, it is more likely to allow the food in your stomach that's being eaten up by hydrochloric acid to come back up ("reflux"), no matter how spicy or bland your meals are. If the walls of your intestines are too stretchy, it doesn't matter how balanced your bacterial microbiome is; your intestines may struggle to push that poop through. This can make you feel like you have sluggish bowels or cause pain because the lax fibers between the muscles allow segments of the intestines to be pushed up where they don't belong.[232]

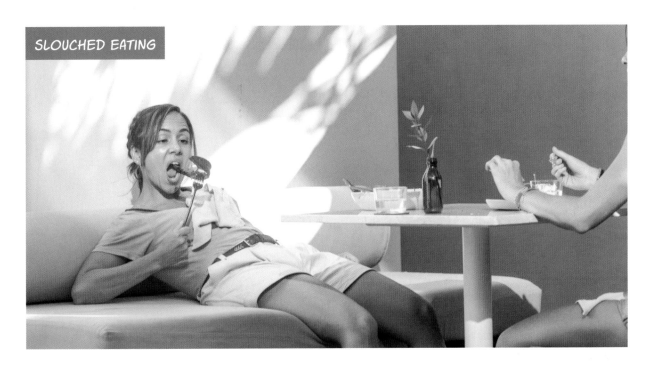

SLOUCHED EATING

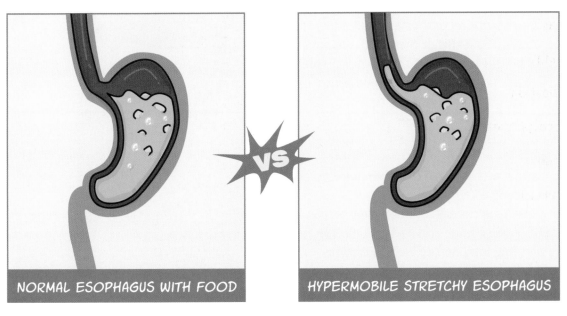

NORMAL ESOPHAGUS WITH FOOD

HYPERMOBILE STRETCHY ESOPHAGUS

Remember the nervous system, too. Poor posture and a lack of spinal stability can lead to dysfunction of the nerves that are responsible for telling your digestive organs what to do.[195] (Refer to Chapter 3.)

Also keep in mind that digestive issues can be totally unrelated to hypermobility. Unfortunately, like anxiety, your gut issues may be a mystery to you for years. But don't see that as a bad thing! View it as a way to listen and learn more about the relationship between your gut and what you eat, how stressed or relaxed you feel, how much and how well you're sleeping or exercising, and, if applicable, where you are in your menstrual cycle. Treat each day as an experiment.

EATING FOR BETTER DIGESTIVE HEALTH

You may be wondering, *What did Adell do? What should* I *do?*

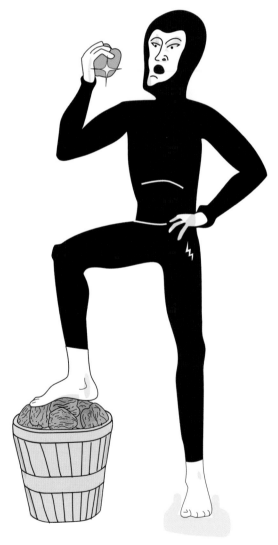

That's a dangerous road, friend. Because if there's one thing you should know, it's that what works for one person may not work for somebody else. You've got to do the work to figure out what is best for you. So you will find no dietary advice in this section. However, there are a few things that benefit pretty much everybody that you can keep in mind and apply to your experimentation.

Unlike the murky and perplexing cause of digestive issues, the solution is (mostly) conveniently simple: eat natural foods in a natural way.

Celest and I are not going to tell you what your diet should look like, or whether you should be a vegan or a carnivore, or if you should add supplements or cut out this or that food. We have our opinions, but we want you to have your opinions, too, and to form those opinions based on your research into which foods make you feel good. We ask only that you look at the foods you eat, the portion sizes, and the frequency and timing of your meals from the point of view of "how different is this from the way my pre–modern technology ancestors would have eaten?"

Our bodies—hypermobile or not—evolved to turn plants, animals, fungi, and bacteria into energy, nutrients, and fuel long before we had endless miles of a single crop that would be deconstructed, refined, and processed in factories and turned into fourteen different ingredients that would go into the perfectly rectangular plastic-wrapped long-shelf-life snacks and meals that fill our fluorescent-lit supermarket shelves.

By that we mean: just eat real food. Whole food. Food the way nature made it. Eat an apple rather than a plastic bag filled with dehydrated apple slices that have been coated with sugar and apple flavorings.

If you don't do so already, start reading the ingredients listed on the packages of food you buy. Develop an understanding of when manufacturers are adding things to make the food taste good, to make you want to eat more, and to make you want to buy more. Yes, it may feel like you're going through a breakup as you realize your beloved cookies don't "feed your soul" but rather trick your brain and body into thinking they're getting a dense energy boost that they can store for later in the form of fat, for times of scarcity that won't happen in your twenty-first-century life. Regardless of the size and shape of your body, the sugars and toxins in those tasty but terrible ingredients may be wreaking havoc inside you, and that certainly doesn't help guard against pain or illness.

Generally, the closer a food is to how nature gave it to us, the better. That being said, cooking makes a lot of foods easier to digest, so pay attention to raw foods that make your apana vayu smell bad and try cooking them instead.[209]

Also pay attention to foods—cooked or raw—that make your belly do weird things (bloating, farting a lot, hurting) and cut back on those. Avoid them for a while and see if it makes a difference in how you feel. Common irritants include:

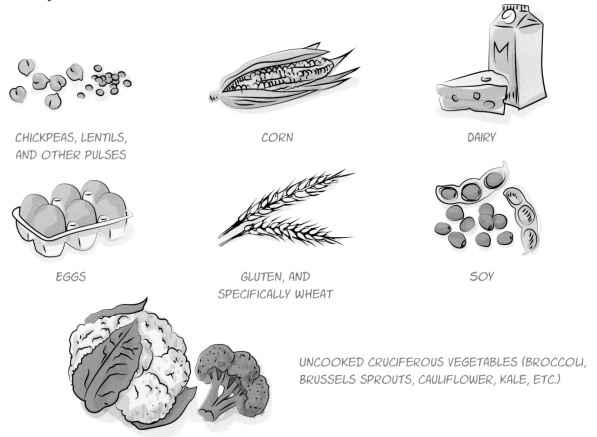

CHICKPEAS, LENTILS, AND OTHER PULSES

CORN

DAIRY

EGGS

GLUTEN, AND SPECIFICALLY WHEAT

SOY

UNCOOKED CRUCIFEROUS VEGETABLES (BROCCOLI, BRUSSELS SPROUTS, CAULIFLOWER, KALE, ETC.)

Some of these things may be superfoods for you. If so, great! Keep eating them. But this is a general list of common culprits to keep in mind.

Breaking Up with Sugar

The food that may be the hardest to break up with is sugar. Back when humans were hairy little bipedal animals hunting and foraging for food, sugar was a rare source of immediate energy. So our ancestors learned to like it and gorged on it when they came into contact with it. But now sugar is everywhere, even hidden in foods that aren't sweet.

If you're new to the information that sugar is really bad for you and your health will improve in every way if you cut back on it *drastically,* then please go do some further research. For this book, we're going to focus on three key facts:

- **Sugar is more than the white powder that covers a donut.** It is honey, maple syrup, and even that apple. It is pretty much anything that tastes sweet. Most natural sugars are a combination of fructose and glucose—that includes both the beloved coconut nectar and agave syrup found in health food stores and the vilified white table sugar and high-fructose corn syrup.[210] It's all sweet. It's all sugar.

- **All sugar is inflammatory, meaning that it causes inflammation in your body.** And inflammation leads to pain—not just gut pain or stomach pain, but joint pain, muscle pain, headaches, and backaches. All these forms of pain could be caused by inflammation, and inflammation is exacerbated by sugar.[211]

- **Sugar is addictive.** If you're used to having a couple cans of soda per day or getting a blueberry muffin with the morning coffee you buy, be prepared to go through some withdrawal. You'll get over it, though.[212]

No, you don't have to cut out all forms of sugar always and forever. You're allowed to treat yourself from time to time, and you're allowed to eat that apple. An apple has benefits aside from the sugar; for example, it contains fiber and vitamin C.[213] Begin to notice the amounts of sugar in the foods you eat and ask yourself if you could replace those foods with less-sugary ones. Just try it. Experiment. See if you feel better without those sodas or blueberry muffins.

Monitoring Your Eating Habits

Finally, it's not only about *what* you eat but also *how, when,* and *how much* you eat. When your body digests your food, it's doing something you probably have no clue how to do: it's transforming that apple or handful of walnuts into fuel. It's breaking down that food into vitamins and minerals and fats and proteins so that your cells can continue to function. That's pretty cool! But it takes a lot of energy.

Because your body has to work hard to digest your food, eating right before bed, for example, might be detrimental to your sleep.[214] Similarly, eating a huge meal that leaves you stuffed like a piñata might mean you're giving your digestive system more work to do than is good for it. So pay attention to your portion sizes and the frequency and timing of your eating. Everyone is different, so that's the end of our advice in this area.

Most of all, pay attention to your eating habits in general. Do you eat on the go? Do you eat while walking down the street or driving your car? Do you fail to chew your food thoroughly?

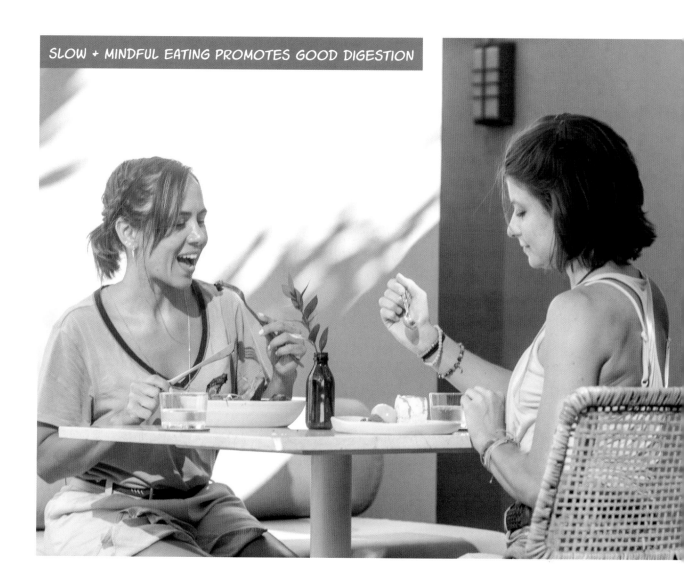

If you answered yes to any of these questions, or if you identify other less-than-ideal eating habits, can you take a moment to take a few slow, deep breaths before you chow down? Then, as you eat, take your time rather than wolfing down your food as though you're in a competition to see who can eat the fastest.[215]

Digestion falls under the parasympathetic nervous system, aka the rest, digest, and repair state. Our bodies digest food best when we're relaxed and calm.[215] So give your digestive system a chance to do its very cool and arduous job.

It may seem too simple to be true, especially in our society, which makes us feel like every solution involves a prescription drug or an elaborate medical strategy that we can't enact without the help of doctors. But actually, just cutting out processed foods and slowing down to eat can do wonders for your gut health.

Your Pesky Gut Is Your Superpower in Disguise

If you deal with digestive issues that normally only people with a horrible diet and lifestyle seem to get, then yes, it could be because of your hypermobility. It's not that you're doing something wrong. It's your *superpower*.

Why is it your superpower? Because you're more sensitive to things than other people. Either you don't know it yet, or maybe you've already figured it out. Maybe you have given up wheat or cut out sugar, and maybe you're more motivated than your friends are not to go so hard on the adult beverages—because you're so much more aware of the consequences, and your digestive system doesn't deal with these substances as easily as others' systems do.

Maybe, just maybe, we are like those dogs that can use their incredible sense of smell to detect cancer in patients. Our sensitivity to slightly toxic foods may give us a viewpoint that others don't have, to sniff out the foods in our modern diet that are harming us all. We feel the effects more stridently, but they're not good for anyone.

Perhaps you will begin to make more of your food decisions based first on whether it will make you feel good and only second on whether it tastes good.

Your Brain and Your Eating Habits

One final thing to remember is, as we've mentioned so often in this book, your brain has to come into consideration here.

If you think about it, the choices you make with regard to eating are, well, less about the actual choices you consciously make than they are the fulfillment of subconscious habitual urges. There's a fascinating and deep connection between how we eat, the emotional ties to our eating habits, and the brain.[225,226]

But that's a whole other book in itself.

We'll just leave you with this tasty food for thought:

If you recognize that you could be—maybe even *should* be—making different decisions about food, but you just can't seem to stick with it no matter how much you KNOW, then remember that your brain is,

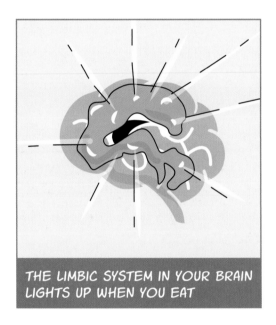

THE LIMBIC SYSTEM IN YOUR BRAIN LIGHTS UP WHEN YOU EAT

well, kinda lazy. It loves things to be efficient and safe, which means it doesn't like change all that much. Change takes energy, and it's risky.

So think less about the food and more about your brain. Give yourself a solid reason for wanting to change your habits. Write it down, say it out loud, tell your friends and family about it. OWN IT, friend!

MY GOALS

_____

_____

_____

_____

_____

_____

_____

_____

_____

_____

_____

_____

_____

_____

_____

_____

_____

_____

_____

_____

_____

Also, tie a positive emotion to your new healthy habit. Even if you don't feel the emotion automatically just yet, fake it till you make it! Tell yourself, "I'm *soooo* excited to eat/not eat this."

Because, Bendy friend, we don't make decisions based on what we know; we make decisions based on how we feel. Over and over again, psychological studies show that in all areas of life, we humans are at the mercy of our feelings over any rationale.

So, hack that!

CHAPTER 13:
HYPERMOBILITY AND FATIGUE

It may come as a relief to hear that if you suffer from fatigue—the kind of fatigue that feels like trying to go for a swim while wearing an Abominable Snowman costume—it may be due to hypermobility.

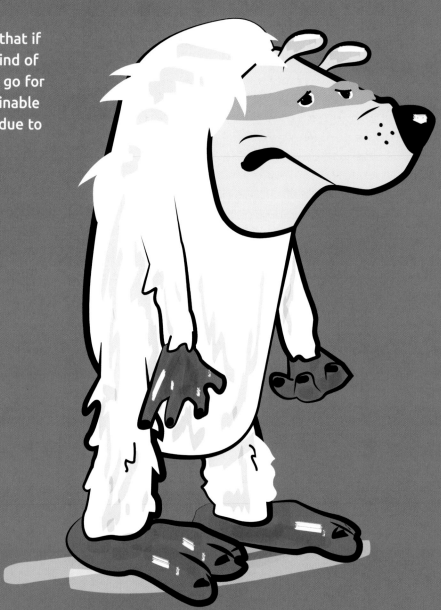

Okay, so that information doesn't offer any cure or treatment, but we feel that simply understanding there's a reason for your fatigue—and that it's not because you're doing something wrong—is therapeutic in itself. But don't worry, we've got some tips for you, too.

POSSIBLE CAUSES OF FATIGUE

Bendies often feel more fatigue, as well as being more likely to have conditions such as chronic fatigue syndrome (CFS), myalgic encephalomyelitis (ME), and fibromyalgia, for the same reason we have more anxiety and gut issues: our extra-stretchy tissues mean that our bodies have to work extra hard! They're doing their best, bless them, toiling away night and day to perform basic, everyday functions such as pumping blood, digesting food, and holding us upright. Just *being* is enough to cause fatigue for some of us.

Insomnia is more prevalent among us super flexible humanoids, too. Even if you're sleeping, you might not be getting a truly restful night's sleep because of churning adrenaline.[198,216] Consistently missing out on good sleep will no doubt have a knock-on effect on everything you, and your body, try to do. If you're not 100 percent on board with us when we say that getting adequate, restful sleep is one of the top things you can do for your well-being, then we highly encourage you to do some research into the importance of sleep.

There's one more really interesting explanation for fatigue (as well as pain and anxiety): it's your brain's way of *making you stop*. With the help of Elastidog (who represents the nervous system), we hope we have made it clear that the nervous system's number one priority is safety.[217,218]

SING IT WITH US! "AH AH AH AH, STAYIN' ALIVE, STAYIN' ALIVE. AH AH AH ..."

Aaaanyways, stay alive is what your brain wants to do above all else! So, if it perceives a threat, it'll do whatever it can to lessen that threat.[218] If Mr. Sloppy, Passive Range of Misery Man, Trendelenburg, or any of the other villains is up to no good and skulking around your house, good old Elastidog will notice before any of your muscular stability superheroes do. Elastidog's response? Fight, flight, or freeze. Most of the time, it's to freeze—to stop.[222,223]

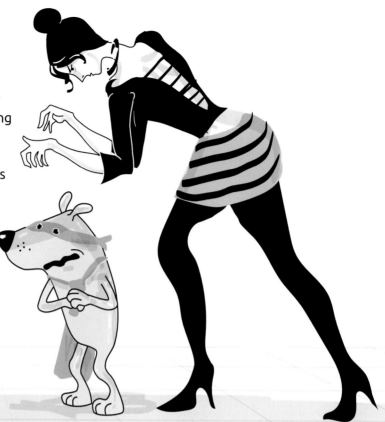

Think of it this way: Once upon a time, you went for a walk and twisted your ankle. As soon as your twisted ankle sent a surge of pain to your brain, what happened? You stopped walking! Elastidog (your brain) remembers this experience. "Hmm, pain makes Bendy stop."

Or perhaps you're once again on a walk, and this time you walk and walk and walk and walk for *soooo* long that eventually you get so tired that you run out of energy. So what do you do? You stop walking! Again, Elastidog thinks, "Hmm, fatigue makes Bendy stop, too!"[223]

So, years later, when you're in a yoga class with the teacher "helping" you get your head between your legs, or you go for a run without bringing Team Gluteus along, or you're really stressed out at work and spending ten or twelve hours chained to your desk and sitting with bad posture, Elastidog remembers. You may not notice it, but Elastidog does.

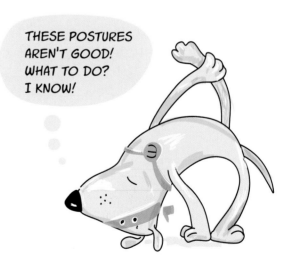

BAM! You get hit by severe fatigue. Or, despite there being no actual tissue damage, you begin experiencing pain. For you, it sucks. But Elastidog is sitting there smugly, thinking, "Danger averted!"

This is why it can be so helpful to understand everything we've written about in previous chapters! When you combine your superhero stability muscles and AROM the Protector with your phenomenal powers, those villains won't come a-knockin' anymore. Elastidog can relax, and you start to feel more energetic and pain-free again.

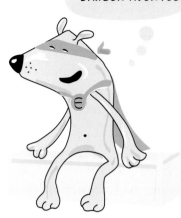

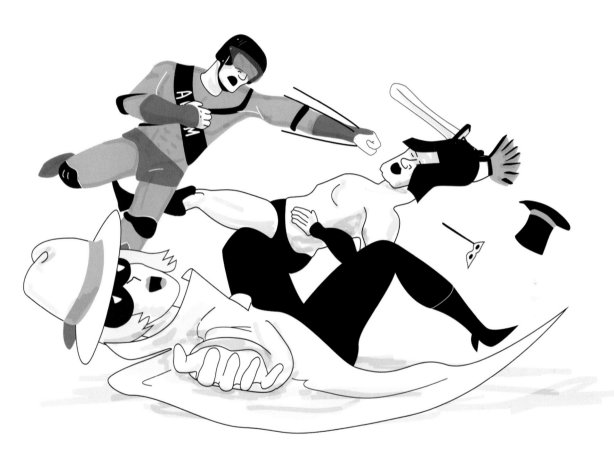

Reading about fatigue could understandably be making your eyelids heavy at this point. If that's you, we totally understand if you want to come back and read the rest of this chapter later. As you'll soon find out, it's super important to rest!

Welcome back. We hope you had a lovely, restful nap. If your mind is hungry for more information about hypermobility and fatigue, then read on!

Too Much Adrenaline

As we discussed in the anxiety chapter, your body may well be producing extra adrenaline in response to the blood pooling in your extra-stretchy blood vessels. With this constant hike in adrenaline, hypermobile people go through activities feeling like they can just keep going and going.[216] Think of the feats people are known to be capable of when they get a sudden adrenaline rush—only to crash with shock afterward.

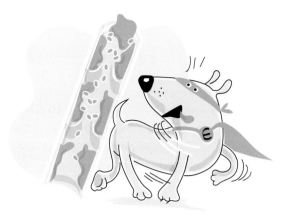

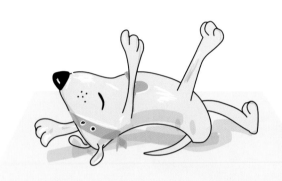

Maybe you've been to a fitness class where the instructor is urging (with all the best intentions), "Don't stop now! I know you've got more to give! Keep it going!" And you, being a star student, think, "Okay, I can keep going! I can push!" Then, after class, you feel like you can barely lift your water bottle to your face to rehydrate from the sweaty workout. Maybe everyone else in the class seems equally exhausted, but unlike everyone else, you don't recover. You go home and lie down on the couch and find yourself unable to move for the rest of the day.

Or maybe you don't need to go to a boot camp class to feel this way. For some of us, merely living life—taking a shower, cranking up the music, and singing a rock ballad into your hairbrush or failing miserably at the shops trying to find a cute outfit for Saturday night—is enough to take you to the doctor to find out what's wrong with you. Your doctor may even have told you that you're fine because your blood tests are normal, or maybe you get a whiff of suspicion from your healthcare provider that you're being a diva or a wuss.

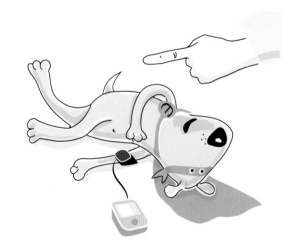

"THAT'S BECAUSE MOST DOCTORS HAVEN'T YET MADE THE CONNECTION BETWEEN ALL OF THIS STUFF!" SAYS CAPTAIN OBVIOUS.

THANKS, CAPTAIN OBVIOUS. WE KNEW THIS ALREADY. BUT YES, YOU'RE RIGHT.

Cervical Spine Instability

Another possible cause of fatigue is cervical spine instability. We mentioned this when we discussed anxiety in Chapter 11 because cervical spine instability can definitely cause anxiety, too. But we'll go a little deeper now.

Cervical spine instability can lead to the compression of the vagus nerve.[19,224] The vagus nerve is, as we've mentioned we like to call her, the momma nerve of the parasympathetic nervous system. There are other nerves that run through that area, too, which are all responsible for the rest, digest, repair, and relaxation part of your autonomic nervous system.

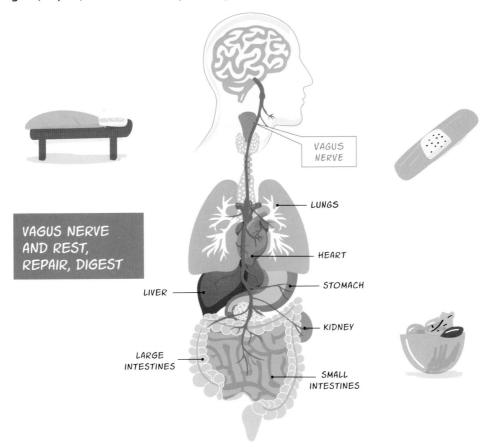

VAGUS NERVE AND REST, REPAIR, DIGEST

VAGUS NERVE

LUNGS

HEART

STOMACH

LIVER

KIDNEY

LARGE INTESTINES

SMALL INTESTINES

So you can think of it like this: some important nerves—the ones that send the "Dude, I'm so chilled out" message—get pressed on if your neck isn't holding your head up properly. That pressure means that the "it's all good" message doesn't get through.

Since Bendy Peeps are especially prone to poor posture in the neck, our chilled-out surfer-dude nerves sometimes end up being muted, mouthing the "Hey man, just relax" signal but not making a sound. If your body isn't receiving that message, then it's more likely to be in a sympathetic state.

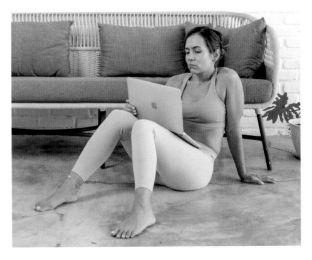

Stress and the Sympathetic Nervous System

And here, the other side, the sympathetic nervous system—the "Hit me! I'm ready for anything!" part of the nervous system—might play a role. Some people who suffer from chronic fatigue syndrome and other severe fatigue-related illnesses trace it back to a stressful event in their lives. Perhaps they contracted a virus that left them sick for weeks while trying to study for exams, or they dealt with the death of a loved one and got a horrible case of food poisoning at the funeral. Something caused them enormous physical and mental stress, and they've never been the same since. The nervous system experienced "stress overload" and relearned a new way to exist: with fatigue. It "gets stuck," so to speak.

The sympathetic nervous system is what enables you to deal with stress.[222] Let's say you finally decide to ask out your crush or tell your boss that you're quitting unless you get a pay raise. Oof, stressful stuff. Your sympathetic nervous system (SNS) may step up, give you some butterflies in your tummy, and say, "Hold my beer. I got this."

This way of dealing with stressful situations such as a job interview or a traffic jam comes from the human body's evolutionary journey through the days of *actual* danger, like running away from predators—perhaps a T-Rex. (We never said this book was historically accurate.) When your SNS says, "Hold my beer, I got this," and you feel that bristling of adrenaline, it means that your body is getting ready to do one of three things:

- **Fight**—because you reckon you stand a chance against that T-Rex if you challenge it to a boxing match

- **Flight**—reasonable if the T-Rex is a bit old and slow, maybe?

- **Freeze**—the "maybe if I stay totally still, the T-Rex won't notice me" strategy[222]

However, if your nervous system gets stuck in that "Maybe if I stay totally still, the T-Rex won't notice me" response, then you may feel like you're locked in a state of hibernation, unable to relax or rest. The autonomic nervous system is malfunctioning, unable to recognize that the perceived threat is gone or never existed in the first place.[222] The result is that the whole body gets overwhelmed by mildly stressful everyday experiences like getting soaked to the bone in an unexpected downpour or tolerating a crying baby on a long flight—things that normally aren't a big deal. But a body stuck in this state *can't* deal.

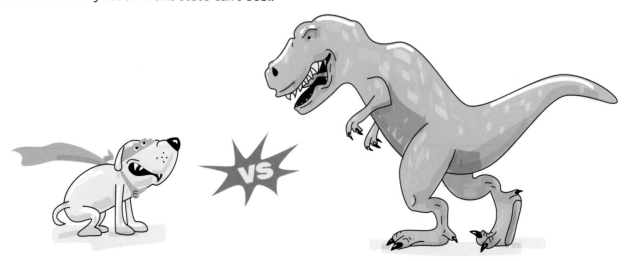

It's also possible to feel like you're always in the state of "freeze." Like pretty much everything else we've covered in this book, that comes down to the nervous system. The simple explanation is that your brain has decided that if it keeps you in "freeze" mode—don't ever move!—you'll be safer. The remedy is to begin to coax your nervous system into feeling safe when you're not frozen.

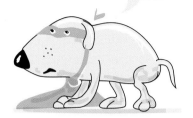

HOW TO COMBAT FATIGUE

Does the kind of fatigue that we've been describing sound like you? Maybe you don't feel such extreme fatigue, but you can think of times when you felt like others around you had a secret for maintaining their energy levels that you hadn't yet found. Either way, here's what to do about it:

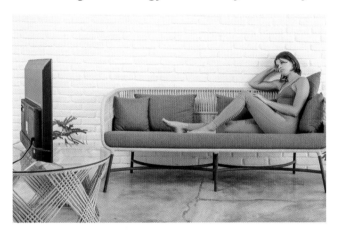

Rest.[221]

Simple, right?

But let's look at what real rest is. It's important to differentiate between "sitting on your butt and chillaxin'" and letting your body go fully into a rest-and-repair state. Have you ever watched a scary movie while sitting on a soft and comfy sofa or had an argument over text messages while lying on your bed? Do you think you were truly relaxed, even if you were reclined on a plushy surface with your muscles at rest?

Achieve True Relaxation

True, deep relaxation is actually mega challenging, especially in our modern world where we are so used to having entertainment and other distractions all around us. If you think *true* rest sounds like anything but the most badass activity ever, then either you've never tried it or you are a relaxation badass already. Because here's the truth: It's way harder than any gym session or yoga class. It takes more discipline than flossing your teeth and remembering to take out the trash.

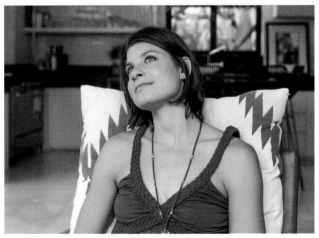

Ask yourself whether you can go without music or a podcast and just be in silence. Answer honestly. Do you ever just sit and stare out the window on a bus journey, or do you always feel the need to be reading a book, scrolling through Instagram, or talking to a friend about the latest gossip?

Sitting still with your eyes closed and simply breathing (you might even call it meditation) is indeed a skill in that it's really, really, *really* hard to do at first. With practice, though, you get better at it. One reason it's difficult is that it can bring up some shadowy thoughts—some darker and more uncomfortable parts of your psyche. It's worth embracing those. Like the night is just as much a part of life as the day, you can choose to see the discomfort of sitting with your shadows as just as much a part of life as the exciting distractions found in the light of day (or the light of your screens).[235]

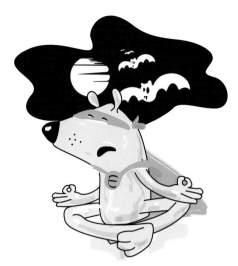

The types of things you can do to help your body relax and recover are the same things that work for other people, but, as a Bendy, you need them more. Here are some suggestions:

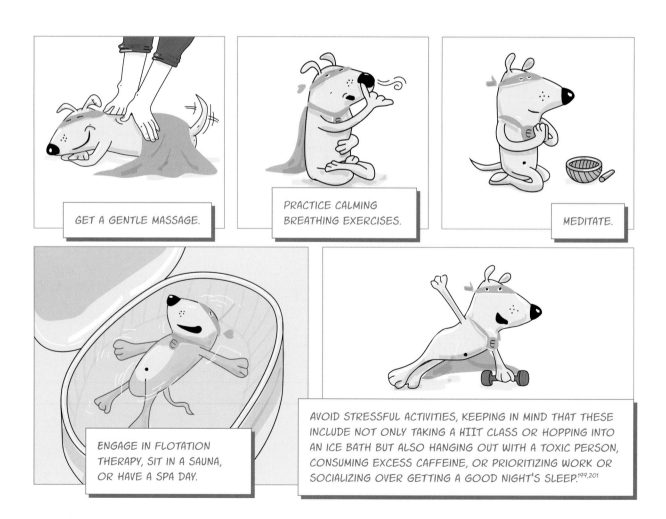

GET A GENTLE MASSAGE.

PRACTICE CALMING BREATHING EXERCISES.

MEDITATE.

ENGAGE IN FLOTATION THERAPY, SIT IN A SAUNA, OR HAVE A SPA DAY.

AVOID STRESSFUL ACTIVITIES, KEEPING IN MIND THAT THESE INCLUDE NOT ONLY TAKING A HIIT CLASS OR HOPPING INTO AN ICE BATH BUT ALSO HANGING OUT WITH A TOXIC PERSON, CONSUMING EXCESS CAFFEINE, OR PRIORITIZING WORK OR SOCIALIZING OVER GETTING A GOOD NIGHT'S SLEEP.[199,201]

EXAMPLES OF CALMING BREATHING EXERCISES[191]

1 Focus on nasal breathing rather than mouth breathing throughout your everyday life.

2 Also focus on diaphragmatic breathing in everyday life; make sure that you're not in the habit of clenching your abdominals and breathing only upward in your chest.

3 Practice 4-7-8 breathing: inhale over a count of four, hold your breath for a count of seven, and exhale slowly over a count of eight. You can exhale through your nose or through pursed lips (the latter can be especially good for calming down from a faster breath). Four rounds take roughly one minute. Repeat as necessary.

4 Practice a pranayama technique called rhythmic visamavritti: inhale for a count of three, hold for a count of six, exhale for three, and hold for six. Repeat as necessary.

5 Practice a pranayama technique called nadi shodhana, or alternate nasal breathing: use the ring finger of your right hand to close your left nostril and inhale through your right nostril; then use the thumb of your right hand to close your right nostril while you release your ring finger and exhale through your left nostril. Then inhale through the left nostril and exhale through the right. Repeat the cycle. You can use the rhythms from the above pranayamas (4-7-8 or 3-6-6-3 counts) or make up your own!

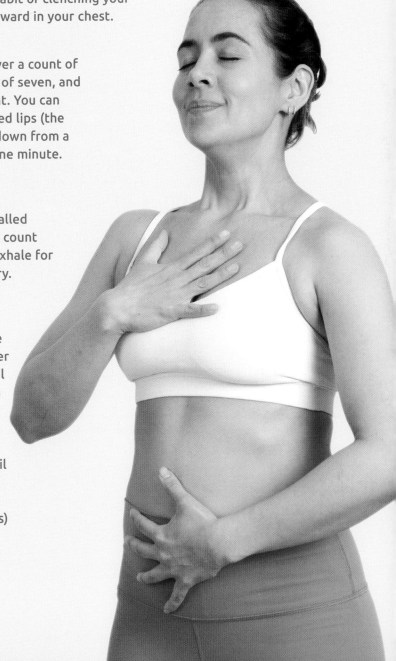

Also, learn to recognize the tipping point when your body goes from "I got this!" to "K, now I'ma need to nap for fourteen hours." You may know that feeling already, or perhaps you still have some learning to do. That's okay! You're not alone—it took Adell thirty-three years of residence in her body to recognize that feeling. Nobody ever explained to her that the feeling that her whole body might be cracking apart or about to shatter was a sign that she was pushing herself too far and needed to stop. "Feel the burn" would turn into "Cry like a baby." She'd be nauseated with sheer exhaustion and have to clear her agenda so she could soak in a magnesium salt bath for the rest of the day. Now she recognizes that feeling and can say, "I need to stop, or I'll crash and burn faster than you can say 'hypermobility.'"

Learning Resilience and Employing Variability

When you feel you have learned this skill of finding total relaxation and you can meditate, breathe, or bubble bath your way to feeling like a baby in its mother's arms without a care in the world, you can begin teaching your body resilience.[219]

Remember progressive overload in training your stability muscles? The same notion applies here. Start with what you can do easily and add on bit by bit.

Being in a sympathetic nervous state and being in slightly stressful situations are normal and even healthy parts of life.[201] It's all about balance. Ideally, you need to be able to go back and forth between "Hold my beer" and "Let's chill out, *duuuuude*" as your present situation dictates.

So you can begin to train this *variability*. You probably already train it in yoga class when you keep your breathing calm and smooth even as the teacher is holding you in chair pose and your legs are burning. Exercise is a form of healthy stress, and, as mentioned several times throughout this book, your breath is the key to staying calm.[220]

Begin to notice when you feel other types of stress, recognizing that some stress, in the right amounts, is healthy and normal.

One way to train variability is to bring focus to your breath and keep it full and even through both cold and heat exposure—for example, going between the cold plunge and the sauna at the spa or switching the tap in your shower between cold and hot water.[202,203]

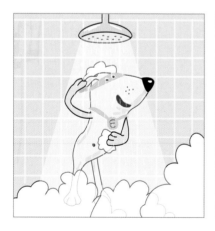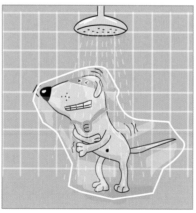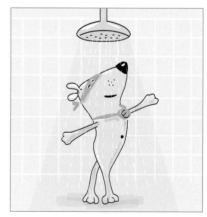

Maybe that crying baby on the plane is a form of stress that you can practice with by tapping into those feelings of calm and peacefulness that you get when you go for a massage or practice pranayama. Recruit that same sense of relaxation when you're feeling triggered by some toxic person.

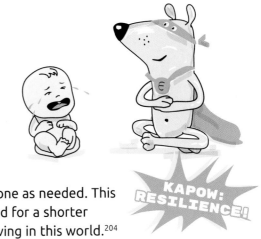

This isn't to say that you should bottle up your feelings and never express frustration or anger. It's more about training yourself to go back and forth between sympathetic ("Hold my beer, I'ma handle this situation") and parasympathetic ("Chill out, *duuuuude*") tone as needed. This will strengthen your ability to be less affected, or affected for a shorter length of time, by stressors that are inevitable parts of living in this world.[204]

HOLD MY BEER, I'MA HANDLE THIS SITUATION.

OR

CHILL OUT, DUUUUUDE.

Finally, when you feel you've pushed it a bit too far and you're struggling to recover, remember the mantra "My body has superpowers." One of those superpowers is that you feel things more acutely than others. You feel fatigue and stress more than others. *This is not a bad thing.* It is your ability to see things that others are blind to and to sense things that others are oblivious to. Like hearing-impaired people can learn to read lips and sight-impaired people can learn to play basketball with an audible ball, your sensitivity to stress just might help you lead a healthier life and be a beacon of healthy choices for others as well.

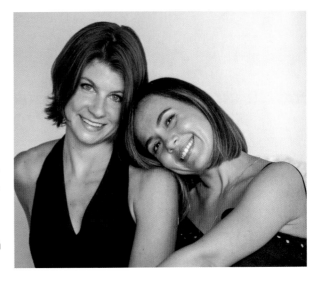

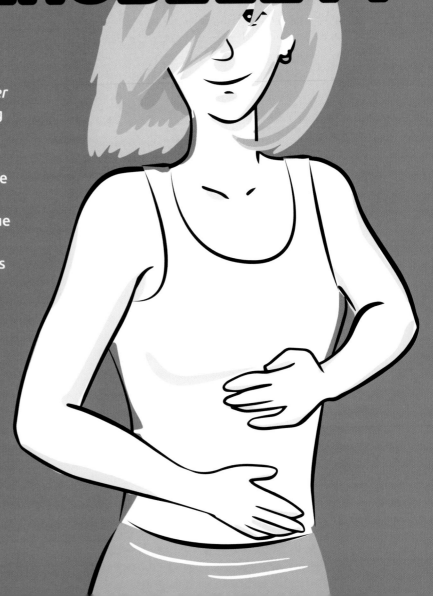

CHAPTER 14:

OTHER PROBLEMS ASSOCIATED WITH HYPERMOBILITY

Other is a dangerous word. *Other* is a word that makes it tempting to oversimplify a complex issue. We hope we've made it clear that just because you might have some kind of pain or illness or condition, it's not necessarily due to hypermobility. For example, you might suffer from gut issues because your diet is filled with foods that your body cannot tolerate, regardless of your collagen structure.

The purpose of this chapter is, like all the other chapters of this book, to shine a light on some possible explanations for the issues you have and suggest some changes you might make to alleviate those issues.

But the work is on you, superstar. The real, hard, transformational work happens when you take this information and apply it day by day to your own unique circumstances, with the mind of a researcher or scientist who's observing their subject without prejudice or preference to understand it better.

With that said, the list of "other" problems associated with hypermobility is long and, according to our research, growing. As medical and scientific researchers give more attention to hypermobility, collagen structures, and the connectivity of it all, the list seems to grow longer *and* wider—longer because there are more conditions on the list, and wider because some of these conditions are now being linked to tertiary conditions that hadn't been connected directly to hypermobility before.

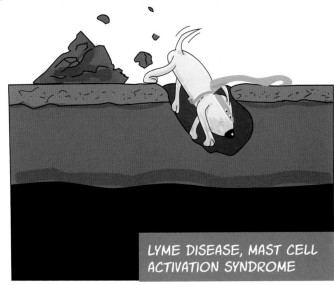

LYME DISEASE, MAST CELL ACTIVATION SYNDROME

Conditions that have been linked to hypermobility include the following:[1,2,3]

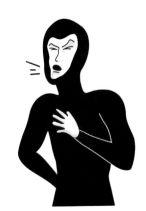

- **Breathing problems**

    - Asthma

    - Improper breathing habits due to poor posture

- **Circulatory problems**

    - Chronic headaches and migraines, like getting a hangover without drinking—definitely a motivator to stay away from binge drinking

    - Light-headedness

    - Low blood pressure (which might impress or even excite your doctors because they see so many people with high blood pressure)

    - Postural orthostatic tachycardia syndrome (POTS)—extreme dizziness not just when you stand up quickly after sitting down for too long but even when you lie down in savasana

    - Raynaud's syndrome, or cold hands and feet due to poor circulation

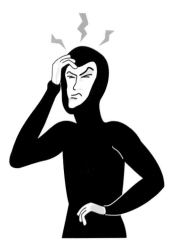

- **Genitourinary problems**

  - Cystocele and rectocele—a form of herniation where parts of the bladder *(cyst-)* or rectum *(recto-)* press into the vagina, causing pain

  - Early-onset incontinence—see Chapter 5

  - Endometriosis

  - Hemorrhoids—varicose veins in your bum hole

  - Interstitial cystitis—a condition in which the bladder may expand too much and not empty totally, leading to infection

  - Ovarian cysts—mostly benign, fluid-filled sacs that can cause heaps of pain

  - Pain during vaginal intercourse

  - Vaginismus—painful spasming of the vagina

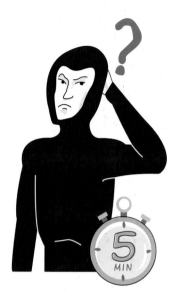

- **Brain differences that affect behavior**

  - Attention deficit disorder (ADD), attention deficit hyperactivity disorder (ADHD)

  - Post-traumatic stress disorder (PTSD)

- **Specific joint problems**

  - Arthritis—joint pain caused by the wearing down of the cartilage between bones

  - Chondromalacia—wearing down of the cartilage in the knees

  - Chronic neck strain—see Chapter 4

  - Costochondritis—inflammation of the cartilage around the ribs

  - Low back pain, bulging discs, or herniated discs—see Chapter 5

  - Neuropathic pain—random burning, itching, shooting pain, or numbness

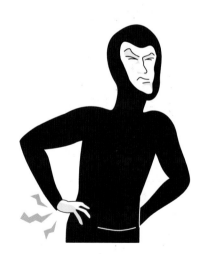

  - Osteoporosis—a disease that causes your bones to become porous, making them frail and more prone to fractures

  - Temporomandibular joint (TMJ) pain—that's your jaw

  - Tendonitis—another word for inflammation in the tendons, which we hypermobile people know all about

- Other digestive problems not mentioned in Chapter 12

  – Acid reflux

  – Delayed gastric emptying—stretchy stomachs don't pass food along efficiently, which disrupts feelings of hunger and satisfaction

  – Overeating—stretchy stomachs that keep on expanding

- Other "other" symptoms

  – Hernias and prolapses—bulges in internal body parts that shouldn't be there

  – Varicose veins elsewhere

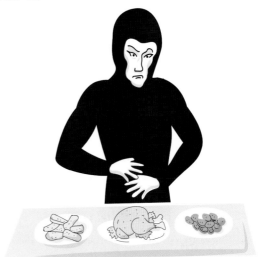

What a bummer.

On the bright side, hypermobile people seem to find labor and childbirth easier. That stretchy tissue comes in handy when a baby is making its way into the world! However, pregnancy also often comes with pelvic girdle pain (PGP), prolapses, and increased lower back and pelvic joint pain.[9]

Major bummer.

Like always, the causes of these conditions aren't straightforward, but a very simplified explanation is that stretchy tissues lead to instability, which leads to things in your body not functioning properly. This shouldn't surprise you at this point, and we can't remind you often enough that everything in the body is connected. So, if your blood can't deliver nutrients to your cells effectively and your nerves can't deliver signals from your brain properly, then that dysfunction will start to take a toll in one way or another.

Fortunately, that whole everything's-connected thing means the solution is pretty straightforward, too. At the time of this writing, our research always comes back to the same conclusion: if we hypermobile people simply look after our health and well-being as we've described in this book—by doing strength training to support our joints, eating well to reduce inflammation, resting fully to allow our bodies time to recover, and remaining vigilant about listening to what makes us feel healthy and strong—then we can harness our superhuman abilities.[8]

It's not a magic pill you can take and then expect everything in your life to get better. That doesn't exist, and even if it did, it would suck. Think about some of your greatest memories and highest highs—they are probably times you got off your ass and did something to overcome a challenge or fix a problem.

Take it from us; there is ginormagantuan (that's even bigger than ginormous) pleasure and satisfaction in developing your glute power and walking down the street one day only to notice, "Oh wow, my back isn't hurting today!" Or how about growing your TVA muscles, which not only helps you feel more solid in your headstand but also finally helps you understand what it feels like to be full after a meal?

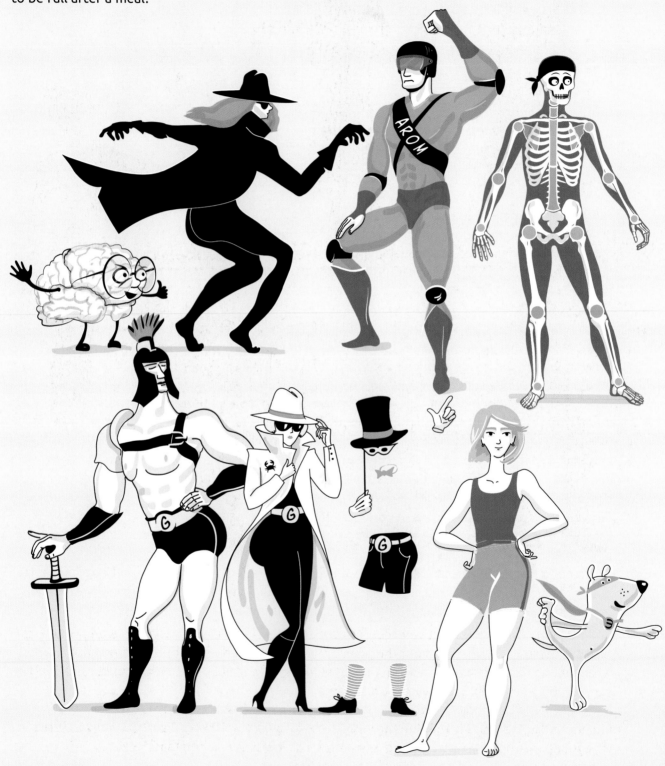

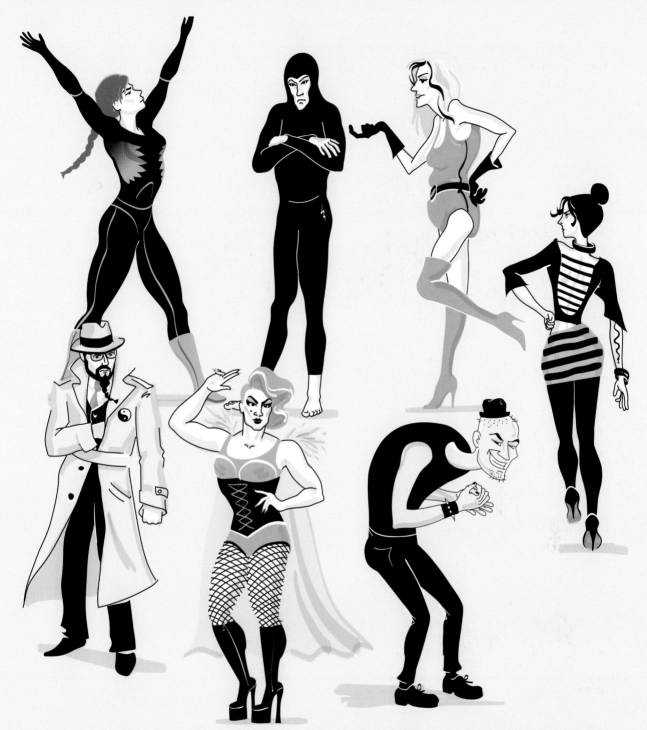

It's bonkers levels of addictive once you start to understand what torquing means in your feet and legs when you walk. If you put the principles we've outlined in this book into practice, you will no longer feel like a humanoid mud puddle oozing through life, but rather like you ordered an upgrade for your body and it was just delivered.

So stick with it, Bendy Friend. Take it from us: there's a whole journey of learning, understanding, letting go, fighting the villains, thinking you're fighting the villains only to learn that your patterns have been getting in the way, learning more, understanding more, and becoming, bit by bit, day by day, a real-life superhuman.

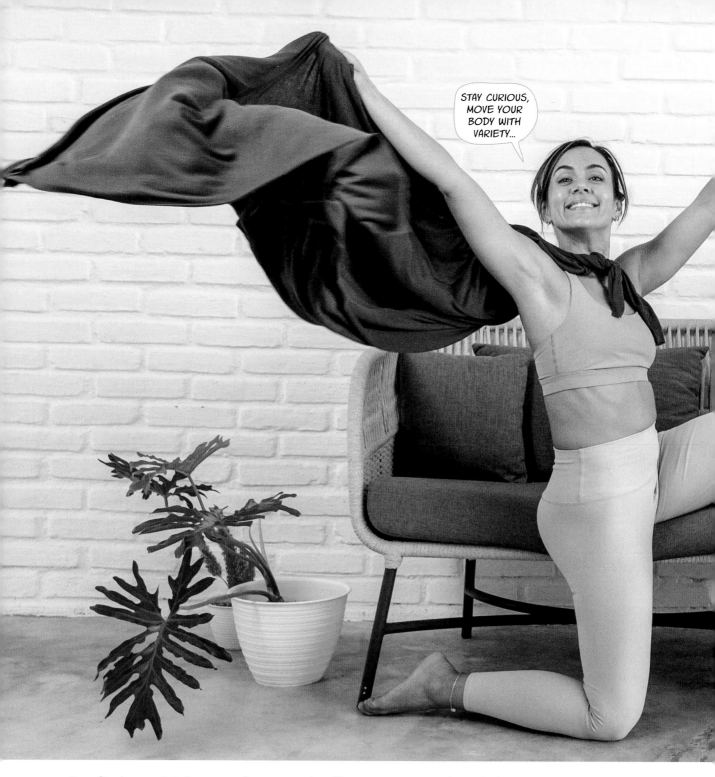

One final note: We know you're a super intelligent person, so this is hella obvious to you, but we wanted to write it anyway: new research is continually shedding light on subjects that were previously hiding in the shadows. While we have done our best to include the most up-to-date information and provide you with the most useful findings, it's entirely possible that while the ink was drying on this very page, a brilliant scientist somewhere discovered something new about hypermobility. Of course, this is the way of the world, so we simply want to remind you to always:

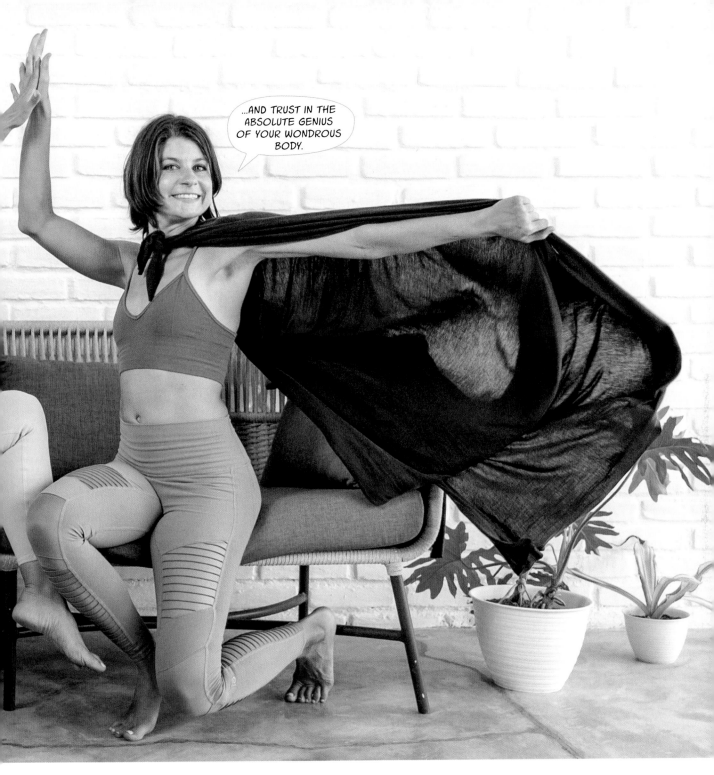

Stay curious.

Move your body with variety.

Trust in the absolute genius of your wondrous body.

REFERENCES

1. Demmler, Joanne C., Mark D. Atkinson, Emma J. Reinhold, et al. "Diagnosed Prevalence of Ehlers-Danlos Syndrome and Hypermobility Spectrum Disorder in Wales, UK: A National Electronic Cohort Study and Case–Control Comparison." *BMJ Open* 9, no. 11 (2019): e031365. https://doi.org/10.1136/bmjopen-2019-031365.

2. Karaa, Amel, and Joan M. Stoler. "Ehlers Danlos Syndrome: An Unusual Presentation You Need to Know About." *Case Reports in Pediatrics* 2013: 764659. Available from: https://www.hindawi.com/journals/cripe/2013/764659/.

3. Simpson, Michael R. "Benign Joint Hypermobility Syndrome: Evaluation, Diagnosis, and Management." *Journal of the American Osteopathic Association* 106, no. 9 (2019): 531–6. https://doi.org/10.7556/jaoa.2006.106.9.531.

4. Radák, Zsolt. *The Physiology of Physical Training*. London: Academic Press, 2018: 119–25.

5. Parvizi, Javad, and Gregory K. Kim. "Chapter 53 - Collagen." In *High-Yield Orthopedics*. Philadelphia: W. B. Saunders, 2010: 107–9. https://doi.org/10.1016/B978-1-4160-0236-9.00064-X.

6. Langevin, Helene M., Maiken Nedergaard, and Alan K. Howe. "Cellular Control of Connective Tissue Matrix Tension." *Journal of Cellular Biochemistry* 114, no. 8 (2013): 1714–9. https://doi.org/10.1002/jcb.24521.

7. Eccles, Jessica A., Felix D. C. Beacher, Marcus A. Gray, et al. "Brain Structure and Joint Hypermobility: Relevance to the Expression of Psychiatric Symptoms." *British Journal of Psychiatry* 200, no. 6 (2012): 508–9. https://doi.org/10.1192/bjp.bp.111.092460.

8. Kumar, Bharat, and Petar Lenert. "Joint Hypermobility Syndrome: Recognizing a Commonly Overlooked Cause of Chronic Pain." *American Journal of Medicine* 130, no. 6 (2017): 640–7. https://doi.org/10.1016/j.amjmed.2017.02.013.

9. Knoepp, Leise R., Kelly C. McDermott, Alvaro Muñoz, et al. "Joint Hypermobility, Obstetrical Outcomes, and Pelvic Floor Disorders." *International Urogynecology Journal* 24, no. 5 (2012): 735–40. https://doi.org/10.1007/s00192-012-1913-x.

10. Bockhorn, Lauren N., Angelina M. Vera, David Dong, et al. "Interrater and Intrarater Reliability of the Beighton Score: A Systematic Review." *Orthopaedic Journal of Sports Medicine* 9, no. 1 (2021): 232596712096809. https://doi.org/10.1177/2325967120968099.

11. Stanton, Tasha R., G. Lorimer Moseley, Arnold Y. L. Wong, et al. "Feeling Stiffness in the Back: A Protective Perceptual Inference in Chronic Back Pain." *Scientific Reports* 7, no. 1 (2017): 9681. https://doi.org/10.1038/s41598-017-09429-1.

12. Jerath, Ravinder, Molly W. Crawford, and Vernon A. Barnes. "Functional Representation of Vision Within the Mind: A Visual Consciousness Model Based in 3D Default Space." *Journal of Medical Hypotheses and Ideas* 9, no. 1 (2015): 45–56. https://doi.org/10.1016/j.jmhi.2015.02.001.

13. Bizley, Jennifer K., and Yale E. Cohen. "The What, Where and How of Auditory-Object Perception." *Nature Reviews Neuroscience* 14, no. 10 (2013): 693–707. https://doi.org/10.1038/nrn3565.

14. Melzack, Ronald. "Pain and the Neuromatrix in the Brain." *Journal of Dental Education* 65, no. 12 (2001): 1378–82. https://doi.org/10.1002/j.0022-0337.2001.65.12.tb03497.x.

15. Tchalova, K., and N. I. Eisenberger. "How the Brain Feels the Hurt of Heartbreak: Examining the Neurobiological Overlap Between Social and Physical Pain." In: Arthur W. Toga, editor.

Brain Mapping: An Encyclopedic Reference, vol. 3: 15–20. Academic Press: Elsevier (2015). Available from: https://sanlab.psych.ucla.edu/wp-content/uploads/sites/31/2016/08/A-87.pdf

16. Watson, Charles, Matthew Kirkcaldie, and George Paxinos. "Chapter 4 - Peripheral Nerves." In: *The Brain: An Introduction to Functional Neuroanatomy*. San Diego: Academic Press, 2010: 43–54. https://doi.org/10.1016/B978-0-12-373889-9.50004-8.

17. Chiel, Hillel J., and Randall D. Beer. "The Brain Has a Body: Adaptive Behavior Emerges from Interactions of Nervous System, Body and Environment." *Trends in Neurosciences* 20, no. 12 (1997): 553–7. https://doi.org/10.1016/s0166-2236(97)01149-1.

18. Schleip, Robert. "Fascial Plasticity—a New Neurobiological Explanation: Part 1." *Journal of Bodywork and Movement Therapies* 7, no. 1 (2003): 11–19. https://doi.org/10.1016/s1360-8592(02)00067-0.

19. Castori, Marco, and Nicol C. Voermans. "Neurological Manifestations of Ehlers-Danlos Syndrome(s): A Review." *Iranian Journal of Neurology* 13, no. 4 (2014): 190–208.

20. Clayton, Holly A., Stephanie A. H. Jones, and Denise Y. P. Henriques. "Proprioceptive Precision Is Impaired in Ehlers-Danlos Syndrome." *SpringerPlus* 4 (2015): 323. https://doi.org/10.1186/s40064-015-1089-1.

21. Mattson, Mark P. "Superior Pattern Processing Is the Essence of the Evolved Human Brain." *Frontiers in Neuroscience* 8 (2014): 265. https://doi.org/10.3389/fnins.2014.00265.

22. Dhabhar, Firdaus S. "The Short-Term Stress Response—Mother Nature's Mechanism for Enhancing Protection and Performance Under Conditions of Threat, Challenge, and Opportunity." *Frontiers in Neuroendocrinology* 49 (2018): 175–92. https://doi.org/10.1016/j.yfrne.2018.03.004.

23. Taylor, Janet L., Markus Amann, Jacques Duchateau, et al. "Neural Contributions to Muscle Fatigue." *Medicine & Science in Sports & Exercise* 48, no. 11 (2016): 2294–306. https://doi.org/10.1249/mss.0000000000000923.

24. Peters, Achim, Bruce S. McEwen, and Karl Friston. "Uncertainty and Stress: Why It Causes Diseases and How It Is Mastered by the Brain." *Progress in Neurobiology* 156 (2017): 164–88. https://doi.org/10.1016/j.pneurobio.2017.05.004.

25. Grichnik, K. P., and F. M. Ferrante. "The Difference Between Acute and Chronic Pain." *Mount Sinai Journal of Medicine* 58, no. 3 (1991): 217–20.

26. Simancek, Jeffrey A. "Chapter 2 - Assessment." In *Deep Tissue Massage Treatment*, Second Edition. St. Louis: Mosby, 2013: 12–25. https://doi.org/10.1016/B978-0-323-07759-0.00007-9.

27. Guido, John A., and John Stemm. "Reactive Neuromuscular Training: A Multi-Level Approach to Rehabilitation of the Unstable Shoulder." *North American Journal of Sports Physical Therapy* 2, no. 2 (2007): 97–103.

28. Storm, Joyce M., Roger Wolman, Eric W. P. Bakker, et al. "The Relationship Between Range of Motion and Injuries in Adolescent Dancers and Sportspersons: A Systematic Review." *Frontiers in Psychology* 9 (2018): 287. https://doi.org/10.3389/fpsyg.2018.00287.

29. Page, Phil. "Current Concepts in Muscle Stretching for Exercise and Rehabilitation." *International Journal of Sports Physical Therapy* 7, no. 1 (2012): 109–19.

30. Luomala, Tuulia, and Mika Pihlman. "Chapter 3 - Physiology of the Fascia from the Clinical Point of View." In: *A Practical Guide to Fascial Manipulation*. Elsevier, 2017: 59–92. https://doi.org/10.1016/B978-0-7020-6659-7.00003-0.

31. Vernon, Howard, and John Mrozek. "A Revised Definition of Manipulation." *Journal of Manipulative and Physiological Therapeutics* 28, no. 1 (2005): 68–72. https://doi.org/10.1016/j.jmpt.2004.12.009.

32. Puentedura, Emilio. "Chapter 78 - Spinal Manipulation." In: Charles E. Giangarra and

Robert C. Manske, editors. *Clinical Orthopedic Rehabilitation: A Team Approach,* Fourth Edition. Philadelphia: Elsevier, 2018: 541–552.e2. https://doi.org/10.1016/B978-0-323-39370-6.00078-0.

33. Ferrell, William R., Nicola Tennant, Roger D. Sturrock, et al. "Amelioration of Symptoms by Enhancement of Proprioception in Patients with Joint Hypermobility Syndrome." *Arthritis & Rheumatism* 50, no. 10 (2004): 3323–28. https://doi.org/10.1002/art.20582.

34. Isenman, Lois. "Chapter 6 - Mental Imagery, Imagination, and Intuition." In: *Understanding Intuition: A Journey In and Out of Science.* Academic Press, 2018: 133–54. https://doi.org/10.1016/B978-0-12-814108-3.00006-3.

35. Shah, Kanishk, Matthew Solan, and Edward Dawe. "The Gait Cycle and Its Variations with Disease and Injury." *Orthopaedics and Trauma* 34, no. 3 (2020): 153–60. https://doi.org/10.1016/j.mporth.2020.03.009.

36. Cai, Liuyang, John S. Y. Chan, Jin H. Yan, et al. "Brain Plasticity and Motor Practice in Cognitive Aging." *Frontiers in Aging Neuroscience* 6 (2014): 31. https://doi.org/10.3389/fnagi.2014.00031.

37. Bø, Kari, Bary Berghmans, Siv Mørkved, and Marijke Van Kampen. "Chapter 6 - Pelvic Floor and Exercise Science." In: *Evidence-Based Physical Therapy for the Pelvic Floor,* Second Edition. Churchill Livingstone, 2015: 111–130. https://doi.org/10.1016/B978-0-7020-4443-4.00006-6.

38. "Ligament Injury and Healing: An Overview of Current Clinical Concepts." *Journal of Prolotherapy* 3, no. 4 (2012): 836–46.

39. Shorter, Emily, Anthony J. Sannicandro, Blandine Poulet, et al. "Skeletal Muscle Wasting and Its Relationship with Osteoarthritis: A Mini-Review of Mechanisms and Current Interventions." *Current Rheumatology Reports* 21, no. 8 (2019): 40. https://doi.org/10.1007/s11926-019-0839-4.

40. Schleip, Robert, Ian L. Naylor, Daniel Ursu, et al. "Passive Muscle Stiffness May Be Influenced by Active Contractility of Intramuscular Connective Tissue." *Medical Hypotheses* 66, no. 1 (2006): 66–71. https://doi.org/10.1016/j.mehy.2005.08.025.

41. Carroll, Timothy J., Barry Benjamin, Riek Stephan, et al. "Resistance Training Enhances the Stability of Sensorimotor Coordination." *Proceedings of the Royal Society of London. Series B: Biological Sciences* 268, no. 1464 (2001): 221–27. https://doi.org/10.1098/rspb.2000.1356.

42. Latash, M. L., and X. Huang. "Neural Control of Movement Stability: Lessons from Studies of Neurological Patients." *Neuroscience* 301 (2015): 39–48. https://doi.org/10.1016/j.neuroscience.2015.05.075.

43. Hoffman, J., and P. Gabel. "Expanding Panjabi's Stability Model to Express Movement: A Theoretical Model." *Medical Hypotheses* 80, no. 6 (2013): 692–97. https://doi.org/10.1016/j.mehy.2013.02.006.

44. Joshi, Shriya, Ganesh Balthillaya, and Y. V. Raghava Neelapala. "Thoracic Posture and Mobility in Mechanical Neck Pain Population: A Review of the Literature." *Asian Spine Journal* 13, no. 5 (2019): 849–60. https://doi.org/10.31616/asj.2018.0302.

45. Park, Se-Yeon, Hyun-Seok Bang, and Du-Jin Park. "Potential for Foot Dysfunction and Plantar Fasciitis According to the Shape of the Foot Arch in Young Adults." *Journal of Exercise Rehabilitation* 14, no. 3 (2018): 497–502. https://doi.org/10.12965/jer.1836172.086.

46. Gross, K. Douglas, David T. Felson, Jingbo Niu, et al. "Association of Flat Feet with Knee Pain and Cartilage Damage in Older Adults." *Arthritis Care & Research* 63, no. 7 (2011): 937–44. https://doi.org/10.1002/acr.20431.

47. Hewett, Timothy E., and Bohdanna T. Zazulak. "Chapter 9 - Rehabilitation Considerations for the Female Athlete." In: James R. Andrews, Gary L. Harrelson, and Kevin E. Wilk, editors. *Physical Rehabilitation of the Injured Athlete,* Fourth Edition. Philadelphia: W. B. Saunders, 2012. https://doi.org/10.1016/B978-1-4377-2411-0.00009-5.

48. DeAngelis, Gregory C., and Dora E. Angelaki. "Chapter 31: Visual–Vestibular Integration for Self-Motion Perception." In: Micah M. Murray and Mark T. Wallace, editors. *The Neural Bases of Multisensory Processes.* Boca Raton, FL: CRC Press/Taylor & Francis, 2012. Available from: https://www.ncbi.nlm.nih.gov/books/NBK92839/.

49. Hallman, David M., and Eugene Lyskov. "Autonomic Regulation in Musculoskeletal Pain." *Pain in Perspective,* October 2012. https://doi.org/10.5772/51086.

50. Booth, John, G. Lorimer Moseley, Marcus Schiltenwolf, et al. "Exercise for Chronic Musculoskeletal Pain: A Biopsychosocial Approach." *Musculoskeletal Care* 15, no. 4 (2017): 413–21. https://doi.org/10.1002/msc.1191.

51. Yilmazer-Hanke, D. "Amygdala." In: Arthur W. Toga, editor. *Brain Mapping: An Encyclopedic Reference.* Waltham, MA: Academic Press, 2015. https://doi.org/10.1016/B978-0-12-397025-1.00232-3.

52. Pailhez, Guillem, Juan Castaño, Silvia Rosado, et al. "Joint Hypermobility, Anxiety, and Psychosomatics—the New Neuroconnective Phenotype." *A Fresh Look at Anxiety Disorders,* September 2015. https://doi.org/10.5772/60607.

53. Purves, Dale, George J. Augustine, David Fitzpatrick, et al. "Chapter 14 - The Vestibular System." In: *Neuroscience,* 2nd Edition. Sunderland, MA: Sinauer Associates, 2001. Available from: https://www.ncbi.nlm.nih.gov/books/NBK10819/.

54. Manto, Mario, James M. Bower, Adriana Bastos Conforto, et al. "Consensus Paper: Roles of the Cerebellum in Motor Control—the Diversity of Ideas on Cerebellar Involvement in Movement." *Cerebellum* 11, no. 2 (2011): 457–87. https://doi.org/10.1007/s12311-011-0331-9.

55. Iatridou, Katerina, Dimitris Mandalidis, Efstathios Chronopoulos, et al. "Static and Dynamic Body Balance Following Provocation of the Visual and Vestibular Systems in Females with and Without Joint Hypermobility Syndrome." *Journal of Bodywork and Movement Therapies* 18, no. 2 (2014): 159–64. https://doi.org/10.1016/j.jbmt.2013.10.003.

56. Borel, L., F. Harlay, J. Magnan, et al. "Deficits and Recovery of Head and Trunk Orientation and Stabilization After Unilateral Vestibular Loss." *Brain* 125, no. 4 (2002): 880–94. https://doi.org/10.1093/brain/awf085.

57. Falkerslev, S., C. Baagø, T. Alkjær, et al. "Dynamic Balance During Gait in Children and Adults with Generalized Joint Hypermobility." *Clinical Biomechanics* 28, no. 3 (2013): 318–24. https://doi.org/10.1016/j.clinbiomech.2013.01.006.

58. Rani, Sahaya, Archana R, and Shyla Kamala Kumari. "Vestibular Modulation of Postural Stability: An Update." *Biomedical Research* 29, no. 17 (2018). https://doi.org/10.4066/biomedicalresearch.29-18-972.

59. Kobesova, Alena, Lenka Drdakova, Ross Andel, et al. "Cerebellar Function and Hypermobility in Patients with Idiopathic Scoliosis." *International Musculoskeletal Medicine* 35, no. 3 (2013): 99–105. https://doi.org/10.1179/1753615413y.0000000023.

60. Milano, Michael T., Lawrence B. Marks, and Louis S. Constine. "Chapter 14 - Late Effects After Radiation." In: Leonard L. Gunderson and Joel E. Tepper, editors. *Clinical Radiation Oncology,* Fourth Edition. Philadelphia: Elsevier, 2016: 253–274.e6. https://doi.org/10.1016/B978-0-323-24098-7.00014-9.

61. Mizumaki, Koichi. "Postural Orthostatic Tachycardia Syndrome (POTS)." *Journal of Arrhythmia* 27, no. 4 (2011): 289–306. https://doi.org/10.1016/s1880-4276(11)80031-1.

62. Ross, Juliette, and Rodney Grahame. "Joint Hypermobility Syndrome." *British Medical Journal* 342 (2011): c7167. https://doi.org/10.1136/bmj.c7167.

63. Garland, Eric L. "Pain Processing in the Human Nervous System." *Primary Care: Clinics in Office Practice* 39, no. 3 (2012): 561–71. https://doi.org/10.1016/j.pop.2012.06.013.

64. Wegener, Stephen, and Mathew Jacobs. "Pain Perception." In *Encyclopedia of Clinical Neuropsychology* (2011): 1848–9. https://doi.org/10.1007/978-0-387-79948-3_763.

65. Giedd, Jay N., Elizabeth A. Molloy, and Jonathan Blumenthal. "Adolescent Brain Maturation." In: V. S. Ramachandran, editor. *Encyclopedia of the Human Brain.* New York: Academic Press, 2002. https://doi.org/10.1016/B0-12-227210-2/00388-5.

66. Nathan, Joseph Alexander, Kevin Davies, and Ian Swaine. "Hypermobility and Sports Injury." *BMJ Open Sport & Exercise Medicine* 4, no. 1 (2018): e000366. https://doi.org/10.1136/bmjsem-2018-000366.

67. Kral, Tammi R. A., Brianna S. Schuyler, Jeanette A. Mumford, et al. "Impact of Short- and Long-Term Mindfulness Meditation Training on Amygdala Reactivity to Emotional Stimuli." *NeuroImage* 181 (2018): 301–13. https://doi.org/10.1016/j.neuroimage.2018.07.013.

68. Mallorquí-Bagué, Núria, Sarah N. Garfinkel, Miriam Engels, et al. "Neuroimaging and Psychophysiological Investigation of the Link Between Anxiety, Enhanced Affective Reactivity and Interoception in People with Joint Hypermobility." *Frontiers in Psychology* 5 (2014): 1162. https://doi.org/10.3389/fpsyg.2014.01162.

69. Taren, Adrienne A., Peter J. Gianaros, Carol M. Greco, et al. "Mindfulness Meditation Training Alters Stress-Related Amygdala Resting State Functional Connectivity: A Randomized Controlled Trial." *Social Cognitive and Affective Neuroscience* 10, no. 12 (2015): 1758–68. https://doi.org/10.1093/scan/nsv066.

70. Vago, David R., and David A. Silbersweig. "Self-Awareness, Self-Regulation, and Self-Transcendence (S-ART): A Framework for Understanding the Neurobiological Mechanisms of Mindfulness." *Frontiers in Human Neuroscience* 6 (2012): 296. https://doi.org/10.3389/fnhum.2012.00296.

71. Krishnakumar, Divya, Michael R Hamblin, and Shanmugamurthy Lakshmanan. "Meditation and Yoga Can Modulate Brain Mechanisms That Affect Behavior and Anxiety—A Modern Scientific Perspective." *Ancient Science* 2, no. 1 (2015): 13–19. https://doi.org/10.14259/as.v2i1.171.

72. Gibson, Jonathan. "Mindfulness, Interoception, and the Body: A Contemporary Perspective." *Frontiers in Psychology* 10 (2019): 2012. https://doi.org/10.3389/fpsyg.2019.02012.

73. Proske, Uwe, and Simon C. Gandevia. "The Proprioceptive Senses: Their Roles in Signaling Body Shape, Body Position and Movement, and Muscle Force." *Physiological Reviews* 92, no. 4 (2012): 1651–97. https://doi.org/10.1152/physrev.00048.2011.

74. Schiefer, Matthew A., Emily L. Graczyk, Steven M. Sidik, et al. "Artificial Tactile and Proprioceptive Feedback Improves Performance and Confidence on Object Identification Tasks." Edited by Manabu Sakakibara. *PLoS One* 13, no. 12 (2018): e0207659. https://doi.org/10.1371/journal.pone.0207659.

75. Adair, J. C., and K. J. Meador. "Parietal Lobe." In: Michael J. Aminoff and Robert B. Daroff, editors. *Encyclopedia of the Neurological Sciences.* ScienceDirect. New York: Academic Press, 2003: 805–15. https://doi.org/10.1016/B0-12-226870-9/01684-1.

76. Degraff, Mathilde, and Holly Battsek. "Use of Weighted Exercise and Gait Training to Improve Function in the Ataxic Patient: A Case Study on a Patient with Acute Motor-Sensory Axonal Neuropathy." *Journal of Medical-Clinical Research & Reviews* 2, no. 3 (2018): 1–3.

77. Salles, José Inácio, Bruna Velasques, Victor Cossich, et al. "Strength Training and Shoulder Proprioception." *Journal of Athletic Training* 50, no. 3 (2015): 277–80. https://doi.org/10.4085/1062-6050-49.3.84.

78. Olson, Carl R., and Carol L. Colby. "Chapter 45 - Spatial Cognition." In: Larry R. Squire, Darwin Berg, Floyd E. Bloom, et al., editors.

Fundamental Neuroscience, Fourth Edition. San Diego: Academic Press, 2013: 969–88. https://doi.org/10.1016/B978-0-12-385870-2.00045-7.

79. Sieb, R. A. "Proposed Mechanisms for Cerebellar Coordination, Stabilization and Monitoring of Movements and Posture." *Medical Hypotheses* 28, no. 4 (1989): 225–32. https://doi.org/10.1016/0306-9877(89)90076-5.

80. Bouvier, Guy, Johnatan Aljadeff, Claudia Clopath, Célian Bimbard, Jonas Ranft, Antonin Blot, Jean-Pierre Nadal, et al. "Cerebellar Learning Using Perturbations." *ELife* 7 (2018). https://doi.org/10.7554/elife.31599.

81. Han, Byung In, Hyun Seok Song, and Ji Soo Kim. "Vestibular Rehabilitation Therapy: Review of Indications, Mechanisms, and Key Exercises." *Journal of Clinical Neurology* 7, no. 4 (2011): 184. https://doi.org/10.3988/jcn.2011.7.4.184.

82. Bliss, Timothy V. P., and Sam F. Cooke. "Long-Term Potentiation and Long-Term Depression: A Clinical Perspective." *Clinics* 66 (2011): 3–17. https://doi.org/10.1590/s1807-59322011001300002.

83. Erkelens, Casper J. "Coordination of Smooth Pursuit and Saccades." *Vision Research* 46, no. 1–2 (2006): 163–70. https://doi.org/10.1016/j.visres.2005.06.027.

84. Hughes, Anna E. "Dissociation Between Perception and Smooth Pursuit Eye Movements in Speed Judgments of Moving Gabor Targets." *Journal of Vision* 18, no. 4 (2018): 4. https://doi.org/10.1167/18.4.4.

85. Franklin, T. C., K. P. Granata, M. L. Madigan, and S. L. Hendricks. "Linear Time Delay Methods and Stability Analyses of the Human Spine. Effects of Neuromuscular Reflex Response." *IEEE Transactions on Neural Systems and Rehabilitation Engineering* 16, no. 4 (2008): 353–9. https://doi.org/10.1109/TNSRE.2008.920080.

86. Yip, Derek W., and Forshing Lui. "Physiology, Motor Cortical." In: StatPearls [Internet]. Treasure Island, FL: StatPearls Publishing, 2020. Available from: https://www.ncbi.nlm.nih.gov/books/NBK542188/.

87. Stokes, Ian A. F., Mack G. Gardner-Morse, and Sharon M. Henry. "Abdominal Muscle Activation Increases Lumbar Spinal Stability: Analysis of Contributions of Different Muscle Groups." *Clinical Biomechanics* 26, no. 8 (2011): 797–803. https://doi.org/10.1016/j.clinbiomech.2011.04.006.

88. Mueller, Michael J Mueller, and Katrina S Maluf. "Tissue Adaptation to Physical Stress: A Proposed 'Physical Stress Theory' to Guide Physical Therapist Practice, Education, and Research." *Physical Therapy* 82, no. 4 (2002). https://doi.org/10.1093/ptj/82.4.383.

89. Rugy, Aymar de, Gerald E. Loeb, and Timothy J. Carroll. "Muscle Coordination Is Habitual Rather Than Optimal." *Journal of Neuroscience* 32, no. 21 (2012): 7384–91. https://doi.org/10.1523/jneurosci.5792-11.2012.

90. Falla, Deborah, Gwendolen Jull, Trevor Russell, et al. "Effect of Neck Exercise on Sitting Posture in Patients with Chronic Neck Pain." *Physical Therapy* 87, no. 4 (2007): 408–17. https://doi.org/10.2522/ptj.20060009.

91. Lynders, Christine. "The Critical Role of Development of the Transversus Abdominis in the Prevention and Treatment of Low Back Pain." *HSS Journal* 15, no. 3 (2019): 214–20. https://doi.org/10.1007/s11420-019-09717-8.

92. Fitzpatrick, Dennis. "Chapter 3 - Phrenic Nerve Stimulation." In: *Implantable Electronic Medical Devices.* Oxford: Academic Press, 2015: 27–35. https://doi.org/10.1016/B978-0-12-416556-4.00003-6.

93. Zafar, Hamayun, Ali Albarrati, Ahmad H. Alghadir, and Zaheen A. Iqbal. "Effect of Different Head-Neck Postures on the Respiratory Function in Healthy Males." *BioMed Research International* 2018 (July): 1–4. https://doi.org/10.1155/2018/4518269.

94. Falla, Deborah, Gwendolen Jull, Trevor Russell, Bill Vicenzino, and Paul Hodges. "Effect

of Neck Exercise on Sitting Posture in Patients with Chronic Neck Pain." *Physical Therapy* 87, no. 4 (2007): 408–17. https://doi.org/10.2522/ptj.20060009.

95. Bordoni, Bruno, and Emiliano Zanier. "Clinical and Symptomatological Reflections: The Fascial System." *Journal of Multidisciplinary Healthcare* 401 (2014): 401–11. https://doi.org/10.2147/jmdh.s68308.

96. Woollacott, Marjorie, and Anne Shumway-Cook. "Attention and the Control of Posture and Gait: A Review of an Emerging Area of Research." *Gait & Posture* 16, no. 1 (2002): 1–14. https://doi.org/10.1016/s0966-6362(01)00156-4.

97. Kim, Jin Young, and Kwang Il Kwag. "Clinical Effects of Deep Cervical Flexor Muscle Activation in Patients with Chronic Neck Pain." *Journal of Physical Therapy Science* 28, no. 1 (2016): 269–73. https://doi.org/10.1589/jpts.28.269.

98. Appelbaum, L. Gregory, and Graham Erickson. "Sports Vision Training: A Review of the State-of-the-Art in Digital Training Techniques." *International Review of Sport and Exercise Psychology* 11, no. 1 (2016): 160–89. https://doi.org/10.1080/1750984x.2016.1266376.

99. Schleip, Robert, and Divo Gitta Müller. "Training Principles for Fascial Connective Tissues: Scientific Foundation and Suggested Practical Applications." *Journal of Bodywork and Movement Therapies* 17, no. 1 (2013): 103–15. https://doi.org/10.1016/j.jbmt.2012.06.007.

100. Krauzlis, Richard J., Laurent Goffart, and Ziad M. Hafed. "Neuronal Control of Fixation and Fixational Eye Movements." *Philosophical Transactions of the Royal Society B: Biological Sciences* 372, no. 1718 (2017): 20160205. https://doi.org/10.1098/rstb.2016.0205.

101. Selkow, Noelle M., Molly R. Eck, and Stephen Rivas. "Transversus Abdominis Activation and Timing Improves Following Core Stability Training: A Randomized Trial." *International Journal of Sports Physical Therapy* 12, no. 7 (2017): 1048–56. https://doi.org/10.26603/ijspt20171048.

102. Hodges, Paul. "Changes in Motor Planning of Feedforward Postural Responses of the Trunk Muscles in Low Back Pain." *Experimental Brain Research* 141, no. 2 (2001): 261–6. https://doi.org/10.1007/s002210100873.

103. Mitchell, Ulrike H., Patrick J. Owen, Timo Rantalainen, and Daniel L. Belavý. "Increased Joint Mobility Is Associated with Impaired Transversus Abdominis Contraction." *Journal of Strength and Conditioning* Research Published Ahead of Print (August 2020). https://doi.org/10.1519/jsc.0000000000003752.

104. Waongenngarm, Pooriput, Bala S. Rajaratnam, and Prawit Janwantanakul. "Internal Oblique and Transversus Abdominis Muscle Fatigue Induced by Slumped Sitting Posture After 1 Hour of Sitting in Office Workers." *Safety and Health at Work* 7, no. 1 (2016): 49–54. https://doi.org/10.1016/j.shaw.2015.08.001.

105. Lammers, Karin, Sabrina L. Lince, Marian A. Spath, et al. "Pelvic Organ Prolapse and Collagen-Associated Disorders." *International Urogynecology Journal* 23, no. 3 (2011): 313–9. https://doi.org/10.1007/s00192-011-1532-y.

106. Faubion, Stephanie S., Lynne T. Shuster, and Adil E. Bharucha. "Recognition and Management of Nonrelaxing Pelvic Floor Dysfunction." *Mayo Clinic Proceedings* 87, no. 2 (2012): 187–93. https://doi.org/10.1016/j.mayocp.2011.09.004.

107. Arjmand, N., and A. Shirazi-Adl. "Role of Intra-Abdominal Pressure in the Unloading and Stabilization of the Human Spine During Static Lifting Tasks." *European Spine Journal* 15, no. 8 (2005): 1265–75. https://doi.org/10.1007/s00586-005-0012-9.

108. Benatti, Fabiana Braga, and Mathias Ried-Larsen. "The Effects of Breaking Up Prolonged Sitting Time." *Medicine & Science in Sports & Exercise* 47, no. 10 (2015): 2053–61. https://doi.org/10.1249/mss.0000000000000654.

109. Aprigliano, Federica, Dario Martelli, Jiyeon Kang, et al. "Effects of Repeated Waist-Pull Perturbations on Gait Stability in Subjects with Cerebellar Ataxia." *Journal of NeuroEngineering and Rehabilitation* 16, no. 1 (2019). https://doi.org/10.1186/s12984-019-0522-z.

110. Green, David A., and Jonathan P. R. Scott. "Spinal Health During Unloading and Reloading Associated with Spaceflight." *Frontiers in Physiology* 8 (2018). https://doi.org/10.3389/fphys.2017.01126.

111. Kim, Eunyoung, and Hanyong Lee. "The Effects of Deep Abdominal Muscle Strengthening Exercises on Respiratory Function and Lumbar Stability." *Journal of Physical Therapy Science* 25, no. 6 (2013): 663–5. https://doi.org/10.1589/jpts.25.663.

112. Chan, Mandy K. Y., Ka Wai Chow, Alfred Y. S. Lai, et al. "The Effects of Therapeutic Hip Exercise with Abdominal Core Activation on Recruitment of the Hip Muscles." *BMC Musculoskeletal Disorders* 18, no. 1 (2017). https://doi.org/10.1186/s12891-017-1674-2.

113. Sapsford, R. R., P. W. Hodges, C. A. Richardson, et al. "Co-Activation of the Abdominal and Pelvic Floor Muscles During Voluntary Exercises." *Neurology and Urodynamics* 20, no. 1 (2000): 31–42.

114. Ghaderi, Fariba, and Ali E. Oskouei. "Physiotherapy for Women with Stress Urinary Incontinence: A Review Article." *Journal of Physical Therapy Science* 26, no. 9 (2014): 1493–9. https://doi.org/10.1589/jpts.26.1493.

115. Herschorn, Sender. "Female Pelvic Floor Anatomy: The Pelvic Floor, Supporting Structures, and Pelvic Organs." *Reviews in Urology* 6, Suppl 5 (2004): S2–10.

116. Sapsford, Ruth R., Carolyn A. Richardson, and Warren R. Stanton. "Sitting Posture Affects Pelvic Floor Muscle Activity in Parous Women: An Observational Study." *Australian Journal of Physiotherapy* 52, no. 3 (2006): 219–22. https://doi.org/10.1016/s0004-9514(06)70031-9.

117. Wallace, Shannon L., Lucia D. Miller, and Kavita Mishra. "Pelvic Floor Physical Therapy in the Treatment of Pelvic Floor Dysfunction in Women." *Current Opinion in Obstetrics and Gynecology* 31, no. 6 (2019): 485–93. https://doi.org/10.1097/gco.0000000000000584.

118. Critchley, Duncan. "Instructing Pelvic Floor Contraction Facilitates Transversus Abdominis Thickness Increase During Low-Abdominal Hollowing." *Physiotherapy Research International* 7, no. 2 (2002): 65–75. https://doi.org/10.1002/pri.243.

119. Hastings, Julie, Jeri E. Forster, and Kathryn Witzeman. "Joint Hypermobility Among Female Patients Presenting with Chronic Myofascial Pelvic Pain." *PM&R* 11, no. 11 (2019): 1193–9. https://doi.org/10.1002/pmrj.12131.

120. Park, Hankyu, and Dongwook Han. "The Effect of the Correlation between the Contraction of the Pelvic Floor Muscles and Diaphragmatic Motion During Breathing." *Journal of Physical Therapy Science* 27, no. 7 (2015): 2113–5. https://doi.org/10.1589/jpts.27.2113.

121. Toigo, Marco, and Urs Boutellier. "New Fundamental Resistance Exercise Determinants of Molecular and Cellular Muscle Adaptations." *European Journal of Applied Physiology* 97, no. 6 (2006): 643–63. https://doi.org/10.1007/s00421-006-0238-1.

122. Franklin, Simon, Michael J. Grey, Nicola Heneghan, et al. "Barefoot vs Common Footwear: A Systematic Review of the Kinematic, Kinetic and Muscle Activity Differences During Walking." *Gait & Posture* 42, no. 3 (2015): 230–9. https://doi.org/10.1016/j.gaitpost.2015.05.019.

123. Huxel Bliven, Kellie C., and Barton E. Anderson. "Core Stability Training for Injury Prevention." *Sports Health: A Multidisciplinary Approach* 5, no. 6 (2013): 514–22. https://doi.org/10.1177/1941738113481200.

124. Buckthorpe, Matthew, Matthew Stride, and Francesco Della Villa. "Assessing and

Treating Gluteus Maximus Weakness—A Clinical Commentary." *International Journal of Sports Physical Therapy* 14, no. 4 (2019): 655–69.

125. De Ridder, Eline M. D., Jessica O. Van Oosterwijck, Andry Vleeming, et al. "Posterior Muscle Chain Activity During Various Extension Exercises: An Observational Study." *BMC Musculoskeletal Disorders* 14 (2013): 204. https://doi.org/10.1186/1471-2474-14-204.

126. Murray, Andrew J., Katherine Croce, Timothy Belton, et al. "Balance Control Mediated by Vestibular Circuits Directing Limb Extension or Antagonist Muscle Co-Activation." *Cell Reports* 22, no. 5 (2018): 1325–38. https://doi.org/10.1016/j.celrep.2018.01.009.

127. MacKinnon, Colum D. "Sensorimotor Anatomy of Gait, Balance, and Falls." *Handbook of Clinical Neurology* 159 (2018): 3–26. https://doi.org/10.1016/B978-0-444-63916-5.00001-X.

128. Felten, David L., M. Kerry O'Banion, and Mary Summo Maida. "Chapter 15 - Motor Systems." In: *Netter's Atlas of Neuroscience,* Third Edition. Philadelphia: Elsevier, 2016: 391–420. https://doi.org/10.1016/B978-0-323-26511-9.00015-1.

129. Stark-Inbar, Alit, and Eran Dayan. "Preferential Encoding of Movement Amplitude and Speed in the Primary Motor Cortex and Cerebellum." *Human Brain Mapping* 38, no. 12 (2017): 5970–86. https://doi.org/10.1002/hbm.23802.

130. Mottolese, Carmine, Nathalie Richard, Sylvain Harquel, et al. "Mapping Motor Representations in the Human Cerebellum." *Brain* 136, no. 1 (2012): 330–42. https://doi.org/10.1093/brain/aws186.

131. Théoret, Hugo, Jasmine Haque, and Alvaro Pascual-Leone. "Increased Variability of Paced Finger Tapping Accuracy Following Repetitive Magnetic Stimulation of the Cerebellum in Humans." *Neuroscience Letters* 306, no. 1–2 (2001): 29–32. https://doi.org/10.1016/s0304-3940(01)01860-2.

132. Synofzik, Matthis, and Winfried Ilg. "Motor Training in Degenerative Spinocerebellar Disease: Ataxia-Specific Improvements by Intensive Physiotherapy and Exergames." *BioMed Research International* (2014). https://doi.org/10.1155/2014/583507.

133. Ivanenko, Yury, and Victor S. Gurfinkel. "Human Postural Control." *Frontiers in Neuroscience* 12 (2018). https://doi.org/10.3389/fnins.2018.00171.

134. Oliveira, Anderson S. C., Priscila B. Silva, Dario Farina, et al. "Unilateral Balance Training Enhances Neuromuscular Reactions to Perturbations in the Trained and Contralateral Limb." *Gait & Posture* 38, no. 4 (2013): 894–9. https://doi.org/10.1016/j.gaitpost.2013.04.015.

135. Cambridge, Edward D. J., Natalie Sidorkewicz, Dianne M. Ikeda, and Stuart M. McGill. "Progressive Hip Rehabilitation: The Effects of Resistance Band Placement on Gluteal Activation During Two Common Exercises." *Clinical Biomechanics* 27, no. 7 (2012): 719–24. https://doi.org/10.1016/j.clinbiomech.2012.03.002.

136. Rathore, Mrithunjay, Soumitra Trivedi, Jessy Abraham, and Manisha B. Sinha. "Anatomical Correlation of Core Muscle Activation in Different Yogic Postures." *International Journal of Yoga* 10, no. 2 (2017): 59. https://doi.org/10.4103/0973-6131.205515.

137. Myer, Gregory D., Adam M. Kushner, Jensen L. Brent, Brad J. Schoenfeld, Jason Hugentobler, Rhodri S. Lloyd, Al Vermeil, et al. "The Back Squat." *Strength and Conditioning Journal* 36, no. 6 (2014): 4–27. https://doi.org/10.1519/ssc.0000000000000103.

138. Sahrmann, Shirley A. "Moving Precisely? Or Taking the Path of Least Resistance?" *Physical Therapy* 78, no. 11 (1998): 1208–19. https://doi.org/10.1093/ptj/78.11.1208.

139. Poehlman, T. Andrew, Tiffany K. Jantz, and Ezequiel Morsella. "Adaptive Skeletal Muscle Action Requires Anticipation and 'Conscious

Broadcasting.'" *Frontiers in Psychology* 3 (2012): 369. https://doi.org/10.3389/fpsyg.2012.00369.

140. Whiler, Lisa, Michael Fong, Seungjoo Kim, et al. "Gluteus Medius and Minimus Muscle Structure, Strength, and Function in Healthy Adults: Brief Report." *Physiotherapy Canada* 69, no. 3 (2017): 212–6. https://doi.org/10.3138/ptc.2016-16.

141. Martín-Fuentes, Isabel, José M. Oliva-Lozano, and José M. Muyor. "Electromyographic Activity in Deadlift Exercise and Its Variants. A Systematic Review." *PLOS One* 15, no. 2 (2020): e0229507. https://doi.org/10.1371/journal.pone.0229507.

142. Evans, Ronald C. "Chapter 10 - Hip." In: *Illustrated Orthopedic Physical Assessment,* Third Edition. St. Louis: Mosby, 2009: 765–842. https://doi.org/10.1016/B978-0-323-04532-2.50015-8.

143. Jeong, Ui-Cheol, Jae-Heon Sim, Cheol-Yong Kim, et al. "The Effects of Gluteus Muscle Strengthening Exercise and Lumbar Stabilization Exercise on Lumbar Muscle Strength and Balance in Chronic Low Back Pain Patients." *Journal of Physical Therapy Science* 27, no. 12 (2015): 3813–6. https://doi.org/10.1589/jpts.27.3813.

144. Brunner, R., and E. Rutz. "Biomechanics and Muscle Function During Gait." *Journal of Children's Orthopaedics* 7, no. 5 (2013): 367–71. https://doi.org/10.1007/s11832-013-0508-5.

145. Takakusaki, Kaoru. "Functional Neuroanatomy for Posture and Gait Control." *Journal of Movement Disorders* 10, no. 1 (2017): 1–17. https://doi.org/10.14802/jmd.16062.

146. Takakusaki, Kaoru. "Functional Neuroanatomy for Posture and Gait Control." *Journal of Movement Disorders* 10, no. 1 (2017): 1–17. https://doi.org/10.14802/jmd.16062.

147. Alshammari, Faris, Eman Alzoghbieh, Mohammad Abu Kabar, et al. "A Novel Approach to Improve Hamstring Flexibility: A Single-Blinded Randomised Clinical Trial." *South African Journal of Physiotherapy* 75, no. 1 (2019): 465. https://doi.org/10.4102/sajp.v75i1.465.

148. Paulin, Michael G. "The Role of the Cerebellum in Motor Control and Perception." *Brain, Behavior and Evolution* 41, no. 1 (1993): 39–50. https://doi.org/10.1159/000113822.

149. Floeter, Mary Kay, Laura E. Danielian, and Yong Kyun Kim. "Effects of Motor Skill Learning on Reciprocal Inhibition." *Restorative Neurology and Neuroscience* 31, no. 1 (2013): 53–62. https://doi.org/10.3233/RNN-120247.

150. Purves, Dale, George J. Augustine, David Fitzpatrick, et al. "Motor Control Centers in the Brainstem: Upper Motor Neurons That Maintain Balance and Posture." In *Neuroscience,* 2nd Edition. Sunderland, Mass.: Sinauer Associates, 2001. Available from: https://www.ncbi.nlm.nih.gov/books/NBK11081/.

151. Goodwill, Alicia M., Alan J. Pearce, and Dawson J. Kidgell. "Corticomotor Plasticity Following Unilateral Strength Training." *Muscle & Nerve* 46, no. 3 (2012): 384–93. https://doi.org/10.1002/mus.23316.

152. Aagaard, Per, Erik B. Simonsen, Jesper L. Andersen, et al. "Increased Rate of Force Development and Neural Drive of Human Skeletal Muscle Following Resistance Training." *Journal of Applied Physiology* 93, no. 4 (2002): 1318–26. https://doi.org/10.1152/japplphysiol.00283.2002.

153. Berman, R. A., C. L. Colby, C.R. Genovese, et al. "Cortical Networks Subserving Pursuit and Saccadic Eye Movements in Humans: An FMRI Study." *Human Brain Mapping* 8, no. 4 (1999): 209–25.

154. Chang, Lou-Ren, Prashanth Anand, and Matthew Varacallo. "Anatomy, Shoulder and Upper Limb, Glenohumeral Joint." In: StatPearls [Internet]. Treasure Island, FL: StatPearls Publishing, 2021. Available from: https://www.ncbi.nlm.nih.gov/books/NBK537018/.

155. Page, Phil. "Shoulder Muscle Imbalance and Subacromial Impingement Syndrome in Overhead Athletes." *International Journal of Sports Physical Therapy* 6, no. 1 (2011): 51–8.

156. Seitz, Amee L., Lisa A. Podlecki, Emily R. Melton, et al. "Neuromuscular Adaptions Following a Daily Strengthening Exercise in Individuals with Rotator Cuff Related Shoulder Pain: A Pilot Case-Control Study." *International Journal of Sports Physical Therapy* 14, no. 1 (2019): 74–87.

157. Roche, Simon J., Lennard Funk, Aaron Sciascia, et al. "Scapular Dyskinesis: The Surgeon's Perspective." *Shoulder & Elbow* 7, no. 4 (2015): 289–97. https://doi.org/10.1177/1758573215595949.

158. Robert-Lachaine, Xavier, Paul Allard, Véronique Godbout, et al. "Scapulohumeral Rhythm Relative to Active Range of Motion in Patients with Symptomatic Rotator Cuff Tears." *Journal of Shoulder and Elbow Surgery* 25, no. 10 (2016): 1616–22. https://doi.org/10.1016/j.jse.2016.02.031.

159. Shitara, Hitoshi, Daisuke Shimoyama, Tsuyoshi Sasaki, et al. "The Neural Correlates of Shoulder Apprehension: A Functional MRI Study." Edited by Gerwin Schalk. *PLOS One* 10, no. 9 (2015): e0137387. https://doi.org/10.1371/journal.pone.0137387.

160. Myers, Joseph B., Yan-Ying Ju, Ji-Hye Hwang, et al. "Reflexive Muscle Activation Alterations in Shoulders with Anterior Glenohumeral Instability." *American Journal of Sports Medicine* 32, no. 4 (2004): 1013–21. https://doi.org/10.1177/0363546503262190.

161. Carroll, Timothy J., Robert D. Herbert, Joanne Munn, et al. "Contralateral Effects of Unilateral Strength Training: Evidence and Possible Mechanisms." *Journal of Applied Physiology* 101, no. 5 (2006): 1514–22. https://doi.org/10.1152/japplphysiol.00531.2006.

162. Marshall, Paul W. M., Haylesh Patel, and Jack P. Callaghan. "Gluteus Medius Strength, Endurance, and Co-Activation in the Development of Low Back Pain During Prolonged Standing." *Human Movement Science* 30, no. 1 (2011): 63–73. https://doi.org/10.1016/j.humov.2010.08.017.

163. Gandbhir, Viraj N., and Appaji Rayi. "Trendelenburg Gait." In: StatPearls [Internet]. Treasure Island, FL: StatPearls Publishing, 2021. Available from: https://www.ncbi.nlm.nih.gov/books/NBK541094/.

164. Hall, M. G., W. R. Ferrell, R. D. Sturrock, et al. "The Effect of the Hypermobility Syndrome on Knee Joint Proprioception." *British Journal of Rheumatology* 34, no. 2 (1995): 121–5.

165. Vleeming, A., M. D. Schuenke, A. T. Masi, et al. "The Sacroiliac Joint: An Overview of Its Anatomy, Function and Potential Clinical Implications." *Journal of Anatomy* 221, no. 6 (2012): 537–67. https://doi.org/10.1111/j.1469-7580.2012.01564.x.

166. Ouchi, Yasuomi, Hiroyuki Okada, Etsuji Yoshikawa, et al. "Brain Activation During Maintenance of Standing Postures in Humans." *Brain* 122, no. 2 (1999): 329–38. https://doi.org/10.1093/brain/122.2.329.

167. Sinam, Vandana, Thonthon Daimei, I Singh, et al. "Comparison of the Upper and Lower Limbs—A Phylogenetic Concept." *IOSR Journal of Dental and Medical Sciences* 14, no. 8 (2015): 14–6. https://doi.org/10.9790/0853-14811416.

168. Shadmehr, Reza, Maurice A. Smith, and John W. Krakauer. "Error Correction, Sensory Prediction, and Adaptation in Motor Control." *Annual Review of Neuroscience* 33, no. 1 (2010): 89–108. https://doi.org/10.1146/annurev-neuro-060909-153135.

169. Keysers, Christian, and Valeria Gazzola. "Hebbian Learning and Predictive Mirror Neurons for Actions, Sensations and Emotions." *Philosophical Transactions of the Royal Society B: Biological Sciences* 369, no. 1644 (2014): 20130175. https://doi.org/10.1098/rstb.2013.0175.

170. Smith, Jo A., Alaa Albishi, Sarine Babikian, et al. "The Motor Cortical Representation of a Muscle Is Not Homogeneous in Brain Connectivity." *Experimental Brain Research* 235, no. 9 (2017): 2767–76. https://doi.org/10.1007/s00221-017-5011-7.

171. Fatoye, Francis, Shea T. Palmer, F. Macmillan, et al. "Proprioception and Muscle Torque Deficits in Children with Hypermobility Syndrome." *Rheumatology* 48, no. 2 (2008): 152–7. https://doi.org/10.1093/rheumatology/ken435.

172. Fatoye, Francis A., Shea Palmer, Marietta L. van der Linden, et al. "Gait Kinematics and Passive Knee Joint Range of Motion in Children with Hypermobility Syndrome." *Gait & Posture* 33, no. 3 (2011): 447–51. https://doi.org/10.1016/j.gaitpost.2010.12.022.

173. Zhong, Yunjian, Weijie Fu, Shutao Wei, et al. "Joint Torque and Mechanical Power of Lower Extremity and Its Relevance to Hamstring Strain During Sprint Running." *Journal of Healthcare Engineering* 2017: 8927415. https://doi.org/10.1155/2017/8927415.

174. Osternig, L. R., C. R. James, and D. Bercades. "Effects of Movement Speed and Joint Position on Knee Flexor Torque in Healthy and Post-Surgical Subjects." *European Journal of Applied Physiology and Occupational Physiology* 80, no. 2 (1999): 100–6. https://doi.org/10.1007/s004210050564.

175. Day, Joseph M., Ann M. Lucado, and Timothy L. Uhl. "A Comprehensive Rehabilitation Program for Treating Lateral Elbow Tendinopathy." *International Journal of Sports Physical Therapy* 14, no. 5 (2019): 818–29.

176. Cooper, Allison, Ghalib Abdullah Alghamdi, Mohammed Abdulrahman Alghamdi, et al. "The Relationship of Lower Limb Muscle Strength and Knee Joint Hyperextension During the Stance Phase of Gait in Hemiparetic Stroke Patients." *Physiotherapy Research International* 17, no. 3 (2011): 150–6. https://doi.org/10.1002/pri.528.

177. Wilczyński, Bartosz, Katarzyna Zorena, and Daniel Ślęzak. "Dynamic Knee Valgus in Single-Leg Movement Tasks. Potentially Modifiable Factors and Exercise Training Options. A Literature Review." *International Journal of Environmental Research and Public Health* 17, no. 21 (2020): 8208. https://doi.org/10.3390/ijerph17218208.

178. Blake, David T., Nancy N. Byl, and Michael M. Merzenich. "Representation of the Hand in the Cerebral Cortex." *Behavioural Brain Research* 135, no. 1–2 (2002): 179–84. https://doi.org/10.1016/s0166-4328(02)00163-8.

179. Verweij, B. H., G. J. Amelink, and J. P. Muizelaar. "Current Concepts of Cerebral Oxygen Transport and Energy Metabolism after Severe Traumatic Brain Injury." *Progress in Brain Research* 161 (2007): 111–24. https://doi.org/10.1016/S0079-6123(06)61008-X.

180. Ackerman, Sandra. "From Perception to Attention." In: *Discovering the Brain.* Washington, DC: National Academies Press (US), 1992. Available from: https://www.ncbi.nlm.nih.gov/books/NBK234148/.

181. Lamp, Gemma, Peter Goodin, Susan Palmer, et al. "Activation of Bilateral Secondary Somatosensory Cortex with Right Hand Touch Stimulation: A Meta-Analysis of Functional Neuroimaging Studies." *Frontiers in Neurology* 9 (2019): 1129. https://doi.org/10.3389/fneur.2018.01129.

182. Russell, Brent S. "The Effect of High-Heeled Shoes on Lumbar Lordosis: A Narrative Review and Discussion of the Disconnect between Internet Content and Peer-Reviewed Literature." *Journal of Chiropractic Medicine* 9, no. 4 (2010): 166–73. https://doi.org/10.1016/j.jcm.2010.07.003.

183. Robbins, Steven, Edward Waked, and Jacqueline McClaran. "Proprioception and Stability: Foot Position Awareness as a Function of Age and Footwear." *Age and Ageing* 24, no. 1 (1995): 67–72. https://doi.org/10.1093/ageing/24.1.67.

184. Salathe, Eric P., and G. A. Arangio. "A Biomechanical Model of the Foot: The Role of Muscles, Tendons, and Ligaments." *Journal of Biomechanical Engineering* 124, no. 3 (2002): 281–7. https://doi.org/10.1115/1.1468865.

185. Zhao, Mingqi, Marco Marino, Jessica Samogin, et al. "Hand, Foot and Lip Representations in Primary Sensorimotor Cortex: A High-Density Electroencephalography Study." *Scientific Reports* 9, no. 19464 (2019). https://doi.org/10.1038/s41598-019-55369-3.

186. Steffen, K., A. M. Pensgaard, and R. Bahr. "Self-Reported Psychological Characteristics as Risk Factors for Injuries in Female Youth Football." *Scandinavian Journal of Medicine & Science in Sports* 19, no. 3 (2009): 442–51. https://doi.org/10.1111/j.1600-0838.2008.00797.x.

187. Sinibaldi, Lorenzo, Gianluca Ursini, and Marco Castori. "Psychopathological Manifestations of Joint Hypermobility and Joint Hypermobility Syndrome/ Ehlers-Danlos Syndrome, Hypermobility Type: The Link between Connective Tissue and Psychological Distress Revised." *American Journal of Medical Genetics Part C: Seminars in Medical Genetics* 169, no. 1 (2015): 97–106. https://doi.org/10.1002/ajmg.c.31430.

188. BBC News. "Yoga: How Did It Conquer the World and What's Changed?" June 22, 2017. Available from: https://www.bbc.co.uk/news/world-40354525.

189. Witvrouw, Erik, Nele Mahieu, Lieven Danneels, and Peter McNair. "Stretching and Injury Prevention: An Obscure Relationship." *Sports Medicine* (Auckland, NZ) 34, no. 7 (2004): 443–9. https://doi.org/10.2165/00007256-200434070-00003.

190. Woodyard, Catherine. "Exploring the Therapeutic Effects of Yoga and Its Ability to Increase Quality of Life." *International Journal of Yoga* 4, no. 2 (2011): 49. https://doi.org/10.4103/0973-6131.85485.

191. Saoji, Apar A., B. R. Raghavendra, and N. K. Manjunath. "Effects of Yogic Breath Regulation: A Narrative Review of Scientific Evidence." *Journal of Ayurveda and Integrative Medicine* 10, no. 1 (2019): 50–8. https://doi.org/10.1016/j.jaim.2017.07.008.

192. Bhattacharyya, Kalyan B. "The Stretch Reflex and the Contributions of C. David Marsden." *Annals of Indian Academy of Neurology* 20, no. 1 (2017): 1. https://doi.org/10.4103/0972-2327.199906.

193. Ahmed, H., and Cairo University. "Effect of Biomechanical Alignment and Jaw Movement on Women with Pelvic Pain." ClinicalTrials.gov. Updated September 1, 2019. Available from: https://clinicaltrials.gov/ct2/show/NCT03740932.

194. Shirley, Eric D., Marlene DeMaio, and Joanne Bodurtha. "Ehlers-Danlos Syndrome in Orthopaedics." *Sports Health: A Multidisciplinary Approach* 4, no. 5 (2012): 394–403. https://doi.org/10.1177/1941738112452385.

195. Breit, Sigrid, Aleksandra Kupferberg, Gerhard Rogler, et al. "Vagus Nerve as Modulator of the Brain–Gut Axis in Psychiatric and Inflammatory Disorders." *Frontiers in Psychiatry* 9 (2018): 44. https://doi.org/10.3389/fpsyt.2018.00044.

196. Thomson, Paula, and S. Victoria Jaque. "Chapter 17 - Performing Artists and Psychopathology." In: *Creativity and the Performing Artist: Behind the Mask*. San Diego: Academic Press, 2017: 281–305. https://doi.org/10.1016/B978-0-12-804051-5.00017-2.

197. Ma, Xiao, Zi-Qi Yue, Zhu-Qing Gong, et al. "The Effect of Diaphragmatic Breathing on Attention, Negative Affect and Stress in Healthy Adults." *Frontiers in Psychology* 8 (2017): 874. https://doi.org/10.3389/fpsyg.2017.00874.

198. Mathias, C. J. "Autonomic Nervous System: Clinical Testing." In: Larry R. Squire, editor. *Encyclopedia of Neuroscience*. Oxford: Academic Press, 2009: 911–28. https://doi.org/10.1016/B978-008045046-9.00653-7.

199. Viana, Ricardo B., Paulo Gentil, João P. A. Naves, et al. "Interval Training Improves Depressive Symptoms but Not Anxious Symptoms in Healthy Women." *Frontiers in Psychiatry* 10 (2019): 661. https://doi.org/10.3389/fpsyt.2019.00661.

200. Richards, Gareth, and Andrew Smith. "Caffeine Consumption and Self-Assessed Stress, Anxiety, and Depression in Secondary School Children." *Journal of Psychopharmacology* 29, no. 12 (2015): 1236–47. https://doi.org/10.1177/0269881115612404.

201. Garfin, Dana Rose, Rebecca R. Thompson, and E. Alison Holman. "Acute Stress and Subsequent Health Outcomes: A Systematic Review." *Journal of Psychosomatic Research* 112 (2018): 107–13. https://doi.org/10.1016/j.jpsychores.2018.05.017.

202. Allan, R., and C. Mawhinney. "Is the Ice Bath Finally Melting? Cold Water Immersion Is No Greater Than Active Recovery upon Local and Systemic Inflammatory Cellular Stress in Humans." *Journal of Physiology* 595, no. 6 (2017): 1857–8. https://doi.org/10.1113/jp273796.

203. Hussain, Joy, and Marc Cohen. "Clinical Effects of Regular Dry Sauna Bathing: A Systematic Review." *Evidence-Based Complementary and Alternative Medicine* 2018: 1–30. https://doi.org/10.1155/2018/1857413.

204. Pereira, Vitor H., Isabel Campos, and Nuno Sousa. "The Role of Autonomic Nervous System in Susceptibility and Resilience to Stress." *Current Opinion in Behavioral Sciences* 14 (2017): 102–7. https://doi.org/10.1016/j.cobeha.2017.01.003.

205. D'Amato, Maria, Antonio Molino, Giovanna Calabrese, et al. "The Impact of Cold on the Respiratory Tract and Its Consequences to Respiratory Health." *Clinical and Translational Allergy* 8, no. 1 (2018). https://doi.org/10.1186/s13601-018-0208-9.

206. Brinkman, Joshua E, and Sandeep Sharma. "Physiology, Respiratory Drive." In: StatPearls [Internet]. Treasure Island, FL: StatPearls Publishing, 2021. Available from: https://www.ncbi.nlm.nih.gov/books/NBK482414/.

207. Tornberg, D. C. F., H. Marteus, U. Schedin, et al. "Nasal and Oral Contribution to Inhaled and Exhaled Nitric Oxide: A Study in Tracheotomized Patients." *European Respiratory Journal* 19, no. 5 (2002): 859–64. https://doi.org/10.1183/09031936.02.00273502.

208. Castori, Marco. "Ehlers-Danlos Syndrome, Hypermobility Type: An Underdiagnosed Hereditary Connective Tissue Disorder with Mucocutaneous, Articular, and Systemic Manifestations." *ISRN Dermatology* 2012: 1–22. https://doi.org/10.5402/2012/751768.

209. Voytyuk, Mariya. 2016. "Increased Energy/Reduced Digestion." *Encyclopedia of Evolutionary Psychological Science,* 1–4. https://doi.org/10.1007/978-3-319-16999-6_2952-1.

210. Mela, David J., and Elizabeth M. Woolner. "Perspective: Total, Added, or Free? What Kind of Sugars Should We Be Talking About?" *Advances in Nutrition* 9, no. 2 (2018): 63–9. https://doi.org/10.1093/advances/nmx020.

211. Della Corte, Karen, Ines Perrar, Katharina Penczynski, et al. "Effect of Dietary Sugar Intake on Biomarkers of Subclinical Inflammation: A Systematic Review and Meta-Analysis of Intervention Studies." *Nutrients* 10, no. 5 (2018): 606. https://doi.org/10.3390/nu10050606.

212. Avena, Nicole M., Pedro Rada, and Bartley G. Hoebel. "Evidence for Sugar Addiction: Behavioral and Neurochemical Effects of Intermittent, Excessive Sugar Intake." *Neuroscience & Biobehavioral Reviews* 32, no. 1 (2008): 20–39. https://doi.org/10.1016/j.neubiorev.2007.04.019.

213. Riccardi, G., and A. A. Rivellese. "Effects of Dietary Fiber and Carbohydrate on Glucose and Lipoprotein Metabolism in Diabetic Patients." *Diabetes Care* 14, no. 12 (1991): 1115–25. https://doi.org/10.2337/diacare.14.12.1115.

214. Kinsey, Amber, and Michael Ormsbee. "The Health Impact of Nighttime Eating: Old and New Perspectives." *Nutrients* 7, no. 4 (2015): 2648–62. https://doi.org/10.3390/nu7042648.

215. Cherpak, Christine E. "Mindful Eating: A Review of How the Stress-Digestion-Mindfulness Triad May Modulate and Improve

Gastrointestinal and Digestive Function." *Integrative Medicine: A Clinician's Journal* 18, no. 4 (2019): 48–53.

216. Domany, Keren Armoni, Sumalee Hantragool, David F. Smith, et al. "Sleep Disorders and Their Management in Children with Ehlers-Danlos Syndrome Referred to Sleep Clinics." *Journal of Clinical Sleep Medicine* 14, no. 4 (2018): 623–9. https://doi.org/10.5664/jcsm.7058.

217. De Wandele, Inge, Lies Rombaut, Tine De Backer, et al. "Orthostatic Intolerance and Fatigue in the Hypermobility Type of Ehlers-Danlos Syndrome." *Rheumatology* 55, no. 8 (2016): 1412–20. https://doi.org/10.1093/rheumatology/kew032.

218. Porges, Stephen W. "The Polyvagal Theory: New Insights into Adaptive Reactions of the Autonomic Nervous System." *Cleveland Clinic Journal of Medicine* 76, Suppl 2 (2009): S86–90. https://doi.org/10.3949/ccjm.76.s2.17.

219. Kwak, Seoyeon, Tae Young Lee, Wi Hoon Jung, et al. "The Immediate and Sustained Positive Effects of Meditation on Resilience Are Mediated by Changes in the Resting Brain." *Frontiers in Human Neuroscience* 13 (2019): 101. https://doi.org/10.3389/fnhum.2019.00101.

220. Childs, Emma, and Harriet de Wit. "Regular Exercise Is Associated with Emotional Resilience to Acute Stress in Healthy Adults." *Frontiers in Physiology* 5 (2014): 161. https://doi.org/10.3389/fphys.2014.00161.

221. Caldwell, John A., J. Lynn Caldwell, Lauren A. Thompson, et al. "Fatigue and Its Management in the Workplace." *Neuroscience & Biobehavioral Reviews* 96 (2019): 272–89. https://doi.org/10.1016/j.neubiorev.2018.10.024.

222. Kozlowska, Kasia, Peter Walker, Loyola McLean, and Pascal Carrive. "Fear and the Defense Cascade." *Harvard Review of Psychiatry* 23, no. 4 (2015): 263–87. https://doi.org/10.1097/hrp.0000000000000065.

223. Noakes, Timothy D. "Fatigue Is a Brain-Derived Emotion That Regulates the Exercise Behavior to Ensure the Protection of Whole Body Homeostasis." *Frontiers in Physiology* 3 (2012): 82. https://doi.org/10.3389/fphys.2012.00082.

224. Maurer, Robert. "Intracranial Venous Sinus Stenting Improves Headaches and Cognitive Dysfunction Associated with Ehlers-Danlos Syndrome Type III." *Biomedical Journal of Scientific & Technical Research* 26, no. 4 (2020). https://doi.org/10.26717/bjstr.2020.26.004374.

225. Ely, Alice V., and Anne Cusack. "The Binge and the Brain." *Cerebrum* 2015 Sep–Oct (2015): cer-12-15.

226. Mathes, Wendy F., Kimberly A. Brownley, Xiaofei Mo, et al. "The Biology of Binge Eating." *Appetite* 52, no. 3 (2009): 545–53. https://doi.org/10.1016/j.appet.2009.03.005.

227. Cook, Gray. "Expanding on the Joint-by-Joint Approach." Available at: http://graycook.com/?p=35. Accessed October 5, 2020.

228. Singleton, Mark, *Yoga Body: The Origins of Modern Posture Practice* (Oxford, England: Oxford University Press, 2010).

229. Faria, Jr., Miguel A., "Violence, Mental Illness, and the Brain—A Brief History of Psychosurgery: Part 1—From Trephination to Lobotomy," *Surgical Neurology International* 4 (2013): 49.

230. Muller, Divo G., and Robert Schleip, "Fascial Fitness: Fascia Oriented Training for Bodywork and Movement Therapies," *Terra Rosa* e-magazine, issue no. 7, https://dl.anatomytrains.com/fascial_fitness.pdf.

231. Bulbena-Cabre, A., and A. Bulbena, "Anxiety and Joint Hypermobility: An Unexpected Association," *Current Psychiatry* 17, no. 4 (2018): 15–21.

232. Pocinki, Alan G. "Joint Hypermobility and Joint Hypermobility Syndrome." 2010. Accessed August 19, 2021. http://www.dynainc.org/docs/hypermobility.pdf.

INDEX

Z